Immune to Fatigue

Healing the Hidden Causes of Tiredness Through Clean Living

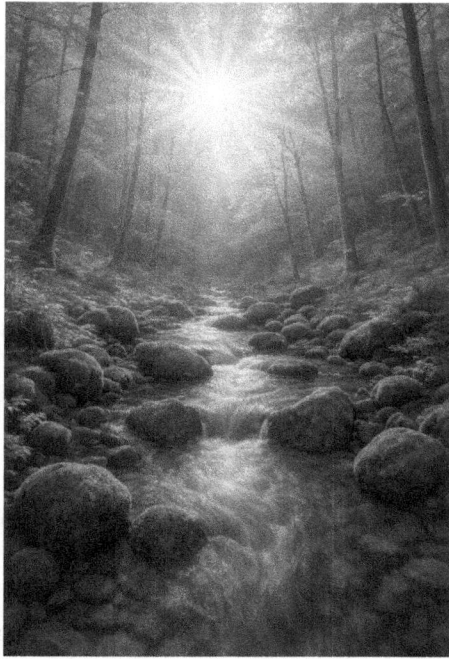

The New Science of Vitality & End of Chronic Exhaustion

Written By: Jesse J. Jacoby

Soulspire Publishing
Truckee, CA, 96161

ISBN: 978-1-968660-28-4
Library of Congress Control Number: 2012921011
Dewey CIP: 641.563   **OCLC:** 213839254

Cover art, font, and layout are all original art by: Jesse J. Jacoby & Abdul Rehman

Wholesalers to book trade: Nelson's Books and Ingram
Available through Amazon.com, BarnesAndNoble.com

Acknowledgements

To the ones who kept me going, and the ones I go on for.

To my children, Arlo and Nevaeh. You are my heartbeat, my daily why, and my greatest teachers. You remind me every day that energy is not a luxury, but a sacred responsibility. I choose vitality so I can show up for you, present, playful, and fully alive. This book is a love letter to your future, and a vow to never burn out.

To the plant-powered endurance athletes. You are living proof that strength does not come from stimulation, but from purity. You have shown the world that plants do not just sustain, they *amplify*. Thank you for running the miles that rewrote the story of what a clean body can do.

To every reader who has ever whispered, *"I am tired of being tired."* I see you. I wrote this for you. I walked this path beside you. Fatigue may have visited but is not who you are. You are light. You are breath. You are power.

To the wisdom keepers, ancient and modern, who taught me to listen to my body, to detox with reverence, to rest without shame, and to reclaim energy as a birthright. Thank you.

To the version of me who refused to settle for survival, who traded stimulation for clarity, and exhaustion for integrity. I honor your choice. You turned your fatigue into fuel.

May this book be a torch in someone else's dark room. May this light the way back to vitality.

Note from the Author

The idea for this book did not arrive in a lab, or a lecture, or a moment of exhaustion. The concept came to me twelve years ago while *mid-stride*, barefoot, with my heart open, and lungs wide. I was sprinting uphill beneath a cathedral of redwoods in Russian Gulch State Park in Mendocino, California.

After years of pushing, crashing, and chasing energy through all the wrong means, I found myself living among the trees. Resting, recovering, and remembering how to feel *alive*. I grew up in Chicago, surrounded by pavement, noise, and pressure, but here, under the silence of the forest canopy, I discovered something profound.

I could run for miles and nothing could stop me. No soreness. No fatigue. No mental resistance. Just rhythm, breath, and endless vitality.

I was eating entirely raw, plant-based foods, juicing greens, fasting with fruit, and drinking clean water. I practiced daily breathwork and slept with the rhythms of the sun. I was living pristine and thinking clearly.

I realized we are not meant to be tired. Fatigue is not natural but is cultural. This is a symptom of disconnection, inflammation, and accumulation. Beneath that weight, though, our bodies hold *a code of endurance*. An ancient blueprint that remembers how to thrive.

That moment in the forest was not just a runner's high. I was experiencing a breakthrough. I remembered that *fatigue immunity* is not a fantasy but birthright. I have spent every day since then exploring how to make this concept a way of life. Not just for me, but for anyone ready to remember their fire.

This book is the path I followed, and now, I offer insights and lessons to you. May these messages reconnect you to your breath, your body, and the brilliance you were born with.

You were never meant to run on empty. You were meant to *run free*.

The Energy Blueprint

Introduction: What If Fatigue Was Optional?

We live in a world where energy has become a luxury, and exhaustion is the norm. Fatigue, once a signal to rest, is now a chronic condition that is misdiagnosed, misunderstood, and medicated. We caffeinate to rise, sedate to sleep, and in between, we wonder why we feel like shadows of ourselves. What if you learned that fatigue is not inevitable? What if the burnout, brain fog, and soul-level weariness so many carry are symptoms not of aging or bad luck but of accumulation?

The truth is that your body is not broken but burdened. Beneath the layers of toxicity, emotional residue, and poor nourishment lies a brilliant, self-healing design. You are not meant to be tired. You are not meant to merely survive your day. The vitality you seek is not available for purchase. This is something you must *uncover*.

We are living amid a silent epidemic. An unspoken collapse of human vitality. From the boardroom to the trailhead, and from classrooms to kitchens, fatigue has become the invisible weight we all carry. Modern medicine offers little more than a patchwork of diagnoses and prescriptions treating symptoms with stimulants and sedatives while ignoring the underlying root. This is a system built on crisis, not optimization. On pathology, not potential.

There is a new paradigm emerging. One that is ancient in wisdom, yet revolutionary in application. *Fatigue immunity* is not a fantasy; this is a biological reality. A natural state that arises when the body is cleansed, nourished, and aligned with original intelligence. When you live in rhythm with nature, and when your cells are flooded with oxygen, minerals, enzymes, and love, you become a being of radiant endurance.

This is not about chasing hype. This is about returning to truth. As Hilton Hotema taught, the body is a temple of light, self-regenerating when free from obstruction. As Thich Nhat Hanh reminded us, peace begins in breath, and fatigue, too, dissolves when we begin to breathe, move, and eat consciously. Additionally, Richard Rudd so often whispers through *The Gene Keys*, true vitality is the result of *alignment* not effort. Energy flows when resistance is gone.

Modern fatigue is not a mystery. This is the predictable outcome of a lifestyle that dishonors the body's design. The result of mucus-forming foods, acid-forming habits, sleep-deprived nights, stagnant lymph, synthetic chemicals, emotional suppression, and overstimulation. We are experiencing the slow drowning of our mitochondria in a soup of toxicity and confusion. The greatest part is that all of this is reversible.

In these pages, we return to the Earth's instruction manual. We explore the ways of endurance athletes like Brendan Brazier and Rich Roll. Not just for performance, but for *presence*. This is not just about finishing races. This is about living a life where you wake up *charged*, connected, and clear.

This book is for the overworked father, the drained mother, the biohacker with a drawer full of supplements and no results, and the seeker who feels like their spark is dim. For anyone who knows that this exhaustion we call *"normal"* is anything but.

Immune to Fatigue is an invitation to shed the weights you were never meant to carry. To cleanse the channels. To trust the brilliance of your biology. To reclaim a state of natural energy that does not fade with the hours but *builds* with momentum.

You were born to be electric, enduring, joyful, and free.

Part I: Understanding Fatigue

Removing the Mystery from Modern Exhaustion

Fatigue is a messenger, not your enemy. A signal and a whisper from the body reminds us that something is out of rhythm. In our world of rushing and numbing, though, we have learned to ignore the whisper, to override the message, and to pathologize the body's intelligence.

What we call *"chronic fatigue"* is often a case of chronic ignoring. A culture-wide misunderstanding of what energy truly is and where energy is sourced. We have been taught to chase stimulation instead of seeking restoration. Mask symptoms rather than address root causes. To measure our worth by productivity, even as our inner light dims.

To become *immune to fatigue* is not to become superhuman. We are simply reverting to being *natural* again. True energy is not found in a pill, a potion, or a power bar. Vitality arises from flow. From unburdened systems. From biological clarity and emotional coherence. When the body is no longer at war with what cannot be processed, we revitalize. When the food, thoughts, environments, and demands no longer exceed our innate design, we can thrive.

Before we can rebuild energy, we must understand what caused the depletion in the first place. This section is about decoding the roots of modern exhaustion. Not with blame, but with compassion. You will discover how the body's energy systems, your mitochondria, nervous system, adrenals, lymph, and more, are impacted by your choices, exposures, and beliefs.

To understand fatigue is to reclaim your power. You stop identifying with burnout as your baseline and start seeing exhaustion as a teacher. As Thich Nhat Hanh reminds us, *"When you rest, you are not doing nothing. You are doing the most important something."* Rest is not a weakness. This is the soil of restoration. Rest alone, though, is not enough. We must also remove what drains us, and feed what sustains us.

Let this part of the journey bring clarity, language, and insight into what you may have felt but never fully named. Let fatigue become the doorway, not the diagnosis. Let us begin to unburden the body, starting with what has been happening at the deepest level.

Chapter 1: The Biology of Burnout

Why Your Cells Cannot Keep Up & How to Set Them Free

Fatigue begins in your cells, not your schedule. Beneath the appointments, the noise, and the caffeine, there is a biochemical orchestra struggling to stay in tune. At the center of all are your mitochondria. These are tiny power plants in every cell of your body, tasked with the miracle of turning nutrients into usable energy.

When mitochondria are nourished, you feel alive. When they are burdened, energy production falters. This is not a matter of willpower or a lack of hustle. The explanation is simple: *your body cannot give what we are not providing through adequate nourishment.*

In ancient traditions, vitality was measured by life force, whether *prana*, *qi*, or *ruach*, but modern science shows us that this force has a tangible root: *oxygen-rich blood, clean fuel sources, efficient cellular respiration, and a nervous system free from constant fight-or-flight.* The so-called mystery of fatigue dissolves when we look at what is really blocking the flow.

Most people are not tired because they are doing too much. They are tired because their systems are clogged, cells are starving, and detoxification pathways are overwhelmed. The body is conserving not lazy. Like a city in blackout mode, the body shuts down non-essential functions to stay alive under the weight of constant strain.

This burden accumulates silently through:

• Refined sugar and rancid oils that smother metabolic fire.

• Pesticides, plastics, and heavy metals that jam up cellular communication.

• Acid-forming foods that displace oxygen and invite inflammation.

• Pharmaceutical residues, synthetic fragrances, and mold toxins that interrupt mitochondrial function.

• Emotional traumas and stress patterns that freeze the breath and lock the body in survival mode.

Then we wonder why the afternoon crashes come. Why we cannot recover from workouts. Why sleep does not refresh us. Why the joy is gone. The answer is cellular repair, not more stimulants. We require oxygenation. We are expected to *release.*

As the Tao Te Ching reminds us, *"To remove that which is not needed is the path of clarity."* When we clear the interference, energy returns. When we purify the bloodstream, rest the organs, and feed the mitochondria with what they recognize, being raw enzymes, electrolytes, structured water, movement, breath, and deep rest, fatigue becomes a memory.

This is not about performance enhancement. You are remembering the baseline you were born with. A body that wakes up *ready*, that recovers quickly, that moves with power and sleeps with peace.

In the chapters to come, we will break down the physiology of fatigue, not in academic terms but in real-world patterns. You will see what robs you, what feeds you, and how to shift the equation. When you stop managing symptoms and start healing systems, you do not just get through the day, you light up from the inside.

The Energy Economy: Why the Body Rations When Overwhelmed

Your body runs on priorities, not preference. When resources are scarce the body begins rationing. This means when oxygen is low, digestion is sluggish, or inflammation is high, the body innately conserves energy for survival. Your immune system slows. Detoxification stalls. Digestion weakens. Hormones fall out of rhythm. What was once a thriving, self-regulating ecosystem becomes a triage unit, focusing only on what keeps you alive, not what helps you thrive.

This is the hidden economy of energy. You do not feel tired because you are broken. You feel tired because your biology has been forced into austerity mode. Think of this like an emergency budget. When income drops, you cut everything nonessential. The same happens inside your cells. Energy that once went toward creativity, libido, skin repair, and athletic recovery now gets funneled toward survival tasks such as basic respiration, blood sugar management, or neutralizing internal toxicity.

In this state, every little stressor costs more. A missed night of sleep. A hard conversation. A processed meal. The interest rates are higher when your energy economy is in debt. This is why so many people feel like they just cannot *"bounce back"* anymore. The bounce is gone because the body's internal reserves are chronically depleted.

You cannot stimulate your way out of this. Energy drinks, sugar shots, and excessive caffeine are loans you cannot afford to take. Each one comes with a crash. A jitter. A crash again. Over time, the interest accumulates: anxiety, adrenal fatigue, liver congestion, mitochondrial exhaustion, and a nervous system locked in constant alert.

You were not designed to push endlessly. You were designed to pulse like waves, breath, and the rhythms of nature. When your life is built on force instead of flow, fatigue becomes your teacher. The lesson is always this: *sustainability is sacred.*

In the chapters ahead, we will begin to restore that sacred rhythm. We will uncover the energy leaks that rob your system and introduce practices that do not stimulate but *build*. These will leave you stronger, not strung out.

The road to fatigue immunity is not paved with quick fixes but is cleared through deep subtraction: subtracting what burdens your body, what clouds your clarity, and what steals your light.

Chapter 2: Tired But Wired

How Stress & Stimulation Hijack Your Energy

A strange paradox of modern life is that people feel exhausted but cannot relax. They lie awake at night with restless thoughts, live with tension in the chest or gut, and yet power through their days on caffeine, chaos, and sheer will. The mind races while the body pleads for stillness. This is the state of being *tired but wired*. A disconnection between appearance and physiology, between outer activity and inner depletion.

This pattern is not just psychological but is also biochemical, hormonal, and neurochemical. Chronic overstimulation from blue light, notifications, synthetic additives, background noise, social pressure, poor sleep, and emotional suppression locks the body in a constant state of sympathetic dominance, known as *fight-or-flight*. In this mode, energy gets diverted toward short-term survival rather than long-term restoration.

You may look *"awake"* on the outside, but your inner systems are screaming for rest. The sympathetic nervous system floods your bloodstream with cortisol and adrenaline, driving up blood sugar, tightening muscles, and causing shallow breathing and digestive shutdown. Over time, this becomes your default mode. An artificial aliveness that masks deep dysfunction.

This state can be addictive. Many people confuse *activation* with *energy*. Caffeine, screen time, sugar, and even conflict can simulate alertness, but these are false fires. They borrow from tomorrow to power today. They give the illusion of vitality while accelerating burnout beneath the surface.

Real energy feels different. There is not just a buzz but a consistent feeling that flows. One that is clean, sustainable, and quiet in power. This allows you to rise early *without an alarm*, focus without strain, and to recover without collapse. What I write of cannot coexist with chronic nervous system dysregulation.

In ancient systems of healing, from Ayurveda to Chinese medicine, energy was not defined by output, but by balance. The yang of movement had to be matched with the yin of restoration. Just as no flame can burn without fuel, no human can sustain motion without restoration.

To move from *wired* to *well*, we must begin to nourish the parasympathetic nervous system. The body's natural rest-and-repair mode. This is the state in which digestion is activated, detoxification flows, hormones balance, and healing begins. This is cultivated not through pills, but through lifestyle: sunlight, breathwork, slow meals, digital silence, earthing, emotional release, laughter, tears, music, and stillness.

To be well also means reclaiming your sleep as sacred. Sleep is not just rest but is also real medicine. This is the time when your brain detoxes, tissues regenerate, and your energy accounts replenish. Yet under the weight of modern habits, most sleep is shallow, fractured, or delayed. We will address this in full in Chapter 8.

For now, pause and ask: *What am I mistaking for energy? Where am I simulating life instead of cultivating?* The difference is subtle, but the long-term cost is not.

To become immune to fatigue, we must liberate our nervous system from artificial demands and provide the opportunity to *remember* what calm feels like. Only then can true, unforced energy rise. In addition to what you do, energy involves what state you are in while you do these things. Every breath, every bite, and every belief either move you toward survival or vitality.

Healing is about doing what matters with rhythm and reverence. This does not require doing more. Build your energy not by speeding up, but by aligning with the natural current.

The Nervous System: Your Inner Switchboard

Understanding the Two Modes of Energy Regulation

Every moment of your life, your autonomic nervous system determines how your body allocates energy through two branches:

1. Sympathetic Nervous System (Fight-or-Flight)

This is the body's stress response system, designed for short bursts of danger, not chronic living.

When activated:

• Pupils dilate.
• Heart rate and blood pressure rise.
• Breath becomes shallow and rapid.
• Digestion slows or halts.
• Blood sugar spikes.
• Cortisol and adrenaline surge.
• Muscles tighten.
• Detoxification and hormone balance pause.
• Energy becomes reactive, not restorative.

Result: You appear *"alert,"* but inside, your body is overclocked, burning reserves, and moving toward exhaustion.

2. Parasympathetic Nervous System (Rest-and-Repair)

This is the body's healing mode, where true energy is built, that is engaged during calm, nourishment, and connection.

When active:

• Pupils return to normal.
• Heart rate slows.
• Breathing deepens into the belly.
• Digestion improves.
• Detox pathways activate.
• Hormones rebalance.
• Mitochondria regenerate energy.
• Sleep deepens.
• Inflammation decreases.

Result: Your body restores, your mind clears, and sustainable energy becomes your natural state.

Checklist: Daily Practices to Restore Parasympathetic Balance

"A rested body is a responsive body, and a responsive body is resilient."

Use this checklist daily to shift your nervous system from sympathetic (stress) to parasympathetic (healing). These simple, consistent habits help rewire your body's energy response toward clarity, calm, and sustainable vitality.

Morning Activation (Without Stimulation)

☐ Rise with natural light (expose skin and eyes to sunlight within thirty minutes).

☐ Hydrate with warm lemon water or mineral-rich juice.

☐ Move your body: rebounding, stretching, walking barefoot, or sun salutations.

☐ Practice 3–5 minutes of deep nasal breathing or box breathing.

☐ Avoid screens and caffeine for the first hour.

Midday Momentum

☐ Take a 10-minute nature break (ideally barefoot or near trees/water).

☐ Eat a slow, plant-based lunch with mindful chewing.

☐ Pause between tasks: take 5 conscious breaths before switching gears.

☐ Engage your lymphatic system: dry brushing, trampoline, or cold bath.

☐ Avoid sugar, energy drinks, processed snacks, and synthetic fragrances.

Evening Wind-Down

☐ Dim lights and avoid blue light exposure after sunset.

☐ Eat a light, early dinner—no later than 7 PM if possible.

☐ Designate a screen-free hour before bed.

☐ Journal or reflect with gratitude (or process emotions if needed).

☐ Enjoy herbal tea, grounding breathwork, and aim for 8+ hours of rest.

Chapter 3: Silent Saboteurs

Hidden Burdens Draining Your Energy

Not all thieves wear masks. Some arrive in invisible forms, being odorless, tasteless, and normalized by culture. They slip past awareness, accumulate in tissues, and quietly unravel the body's energy systems over time. These are the silent saboteurs. If you have been *"doing everything right"* but still feel tired, this is where to look.

Fatigue is often not about what is missing but about what is *blocking*. You may be eating the right food, exercising, and even sleeping well, but if your body is carrying an invisible toxic load, energy will remain elusive. Mitochondria, the energy generators in your cells, are especially sensitive to these stressors. When burdened, they downregulate output. This is a form of protection, not punishment.

The Toxic Accumulation Nobody Talks About

Modern life exposes us to thousands of synthetic chemicals the body was never designed to process.

These include:

• Pesticides in produce.
• Herbicides in lawns and parks.
• Flame retardants in furniture.
• Microplastics in food and water.
• Heavy metals in fish, fillings, and vaccines.
• VOCs in paints, new clothes, and cleaning agents.
• Synthetic fragrances in detergents, perfumes, and air fresheners.

Each exposure might seem small, but over time, they saturate our tissues, disrupt enzymes, mimic hormones, and confuse the immune system. Fatigue is one of the first red flags. Not illness or disease. Just the slow fade of your spark.

Still, we normalize this, saying, *"Everyone is tired. That is just life."* The truth is, what we are experiencing is the result of unexamined burden, not just life. This is a body asking to be emptied.

Mold, Parasites, and Low-Grade Infections

Other saboteurs live inside us. Mold exposure, particularly from water-damaged buildings, is one of the most overlooked causes of chronic fatigue. Mycotoxins can inflame the brain, impair oxygen transport, and damage mitochondria. Some people live for years with fatigue, brain fog, or anxiety, never realizing their walls are quietly poisoning them.

Parasites, too, are more common than we think. Especially in those with weak digestion, poor bile flow, or prior antibiotic use. These unwelcome guests steal nutrients, create toxic byproducts, and suppress immunity, leaving you inflamed and exhausted without knowing why.

Low-grade infections such as Epstein-Barr virus (EBV), Lyme co-infections, or candida overgrowth may also linger below the threshold of medical diagnosis but drain the body, nonetheless. The immune system stays slightly activated, like a light left on in every room. Over time, this all adds up.

The Electromagnetic Cloud

We are electric beings. Every cell communicates through voltage, frequency, and light. So, this is no surprise that our modern soup of EMFs from Wi-Fi, 5G, Bluetooth, and smart meters can dysregulate our energy field. For some, the effects are subtle: *poor sleep, low mood, sluggish mornings.* For others, this can be profound: *migraines, anxiety, or a complete collapse of vitality.*

While science is still catching up, the human nervous system already knows. We are informed with headaches, muscle tension, and that subtle sense of unease we feel when surrounded by artificial frequency with no space to ground.

The Body Remembers What Cannot Be Processed

You may not remember your exposures, but your body does. Toxins, parasites, and frequencies leave energetic and biochemical imprints. Until they are cleared, the body must work harder to maintain baseline function.

The path to fatigue immunity involves subtracting what does not belong, not adding more in. When we clear the mold, the metals, the parasites, and the EMF overload, something remarkable happens: the body begins to hum again. The mind sharpens. The skin glows. The breath deepens. Then, energy that is clean, natural, and grounded returns like a familiar friend.

Top 10 Hidden Fatigue Triggers

These common yet overlooked exposures drain your energy from the inside out. Each one interferes with cellular function, disrupts hormones, or burdens detoxification pathways, leading to chronic exhaustion.

1. Mold Mycotoxins
Found in water-damaged buildings, carpets, drywall, or AC units. Impairs mitochondrial respiration and oxygen transport.

2. Heavy Metals
Mercury (from fillings & fish), aluminum (from deodorants & cookware), and lead (in old pipes or paint) disrupt enzymes and deplete antioxidants.

3. Glyphosate & Pesticides
Common in non-organic produce and grains. Damages gut lining, microbiome diversity, and hormone function.

4. Synthetic Fragrances
Air fresheners, candles, detergents, perfumes. These contain hormone-disrupting phthalates and VOCs that strain the liver.

5. EMF Radiation
From Wi-Fi routers, Bluetooth devices, smart meters, and 5G towers. Alters cellular voltage and nervous system regulation.

6. Parasites
Hidden infections that steal nutrients, create inflammation, and interfere with detox processes. Common after antibiotics or travel.

7. Candida Overgrowth
Fungal imbalance in the gut that produces toxins like acetaldehyde is linked to brain fog and fatigue.

8. Food Additives
MSG, artificial sweeteners, dyes, and preservatives can each trigger immune reactions and neurologic depletion.

9. Tap Water Contaminants
Fluoride, chlorine, microplastics, and pharmaceutical residues all burden detoxification systems daily.

10. Emotional Suppression
Unprocessed trauma, grief, or stress becomes somatic weight, often manifesting as chronic tension and deep fatigue.

Toxin Audit: How to Spot the Invisible Burdens

A Self-Assessment Checklist

Use this audit to assess potential hidden exposures contributing to your fatigue. Check all that apply.

Home Environment

☐ I have lived or worked in a water-damaged building.

☐ I notice musty smells or condensation on windows.

☐ I use air fresheners, candles, or scented laundry products.

☐ I sleep near a Wi-Fi router or smart meter.

☐ My house has old paint, pipes, or carpeting.

Food & Water

☐ I frequently eat non-organic produce or factory-farmed meat.

☐ I use tap water without a high-quality filter.

☐ I consume processed snacks, flavored drinks, or fast food.

☐ I have dental amalgam (mercury) fillings.

☐ I use aluminum-based cookware or foil regularly.

Body & Lifestyle

☐ I use conventional deodorants, lotions, or perfumes.

☐ I have taken antibiotics multiple times in my life.

☐ I experience bloating, brain fog, or frequent fatigue.

☐ I have never done a parasite cleanse or heavy metal detox.

☐ I feel tired even after "sleeping enough."

Scoring Guidance:

If you checked five or more boxes, your body is likely carrying an invisible toxic load.

If you checked 8 or more, this indicates the time for you to begin gentle detoxification and nervous system reset protocols.

Part II: Detoxify Your Energy Pathways

Clearing the Blockages That Dull Your Spark

Once you have seen what burdens you, the next step is to begin *releasing*. Fatigue is not always a signal of deficiency. Often this is a sign of congestion. The body is not tired from being incapable. Tiredness comes from being *clogged*. Energy wants to move, and vitality wants to rise, but blocked pathways and overwhelmed systems act like traffic jams within your biology, slowing everything down.

The promise of detoxification is not found in a quick juice cleanse or a bottle labeled *"cleanse."* Detox is not an event. This is a biological *process*. One that happens every second in your liver, colon, kidneys, lymph, skin, and lungs. When those systems are supported, your natural energy returns. Not as a spike, but as a steady flame.

Modern life throws too much at the body, and while we cannot avoid all exposure, we *can* open the exits. We can clear the channels. We can remind the body there is safety in letting go. When we do release, clarity returns, digestion improves, the breath deepens, and fatigue begins to fade.

To detox is to *unburden*. To unburden is to return to your natural rhythm. This part of the journey will walk you through the practical, powerful practices that support the body's excretory and regulatory systems. You will learn how to gently assist the liver, reignite lymphatic flow, clear the colon, mobilize stagnation in the tissues, and release years of stored waste – physically, emotionally, and energetically.

In the words of an old Taoist proverb: *"The body knows how to heal when the path is clear."*

Chapter 4: Clear the Channels

Opening the Pathways of Detoxification

You simply cannot be energized if you are congested. Vitality is not something you add to the body. This *emerges* when the waste is removed. Just as a river regains her current when debris is cleared, your body regains flow when detoxification channels are open.

There are six primary elimination pathways in the body: colon, liver, kidneys, lymphatic system, lungs, and skin. When one becomes stagnant, others compensate. When multiple paths are blocked, the body has no safe way to offload internal burden, and this burden becomes fatigue, inflammation, and dysfunction.

In truth, most people are not *toxic* because they live recklessly, they are toxic because they are *retaining*. The exits are blocked. Their bodies are doing the best they can under the weight of decades of slow elimination.

The Colon: The Final Exit

If the colon is sluggish, everything backs up. This is the body's sewage system. When not emptied fully and regularly, toxins reabsorb into the bloodstream. This creates a cycle of autointoxication: *fatigue, fogginess, breakouts, bloating, poor nutrient absorption, and even mood disorders.*

A clean colon is the first step toward a clean life. Daily bowel movements are essential. not just for digestion but for overall energy. Raw fruits, fiber-rich plants, magnesium, enemas, and colon hydrotherapy can restore regularity and remove years of compacted waste.

The Liver: Master Alchemist of Toxins

Your liver filters every drop of blood in your body every three minutes. This organ metabolizes hormones, neutralizes chemicals, and transforms toxins for safe elimination. In the modern world, though, our liver is often overworked and under-loved.

Signs of a sluggish liver include: fatigue after eating, irritability, hormone imbalance, and intolerance to fats or alcohol. Support your liver with bitter greens, dandelion root, milk thistle, turmeric, castor oil packs, and lemon water. Light, plant-based eating gives the liver room to *breathe* and renew.

The Kidneys: Silent Filters of Life Force

The kidneys regulate water, electrolytes, and blood pressure, and remove acid-forming wastes. When overloaded with animal proteins, caffeine, or dehydration, they lose efficiency.

Support comes through pure hydration. This can be obtained from structured water, raw juices, and herbal teas like nettle or parsley. Eliminate excess sodium and embrace high-potassium foods like coconut water, watermelon, cucumber, and leafy greens.

The Lymph: Your Forgotten River

Unlike blood, your lymphatic system has no pump and relies entirely on movement, breath, and muscle contraction to circulate and drain. If the lymph is stagnant, toxins and cellular debris remain trapped in tissues, leading to fatigue, swelling, fogginess, and even anxiety.

To move lymph: jump, walk, bounce, and breathe deep. Use dry brushing, sauna, contrast showers, and lymphatic massage. Avoid restrictive clothing and sit less. Lymph is movement, so move.

Kambo is an excellent alternative treatment for regenerating lymph.

The Lungs: Breath as Filter & Fuel

Your lungs not only bring oxygen, but they also release waste in the form of carbon dioxide. Shallow breathing traps tension and limits cellular oxygenation. Without breath, there is no vitality.

Practice nasal breathing, breath holds, diaphragmatic expansion, and breathwork techniques that help you purge and energize. Clean air matters too. Open windows, use air purifiers, and avoid synthetic scents and mold-prone spaces.

The Skin: Your Third Kidney

When other detox pathways are overwhelmed, the skin steps in. This can show up as rashes, acne, or body odor. These are all signs that internal waste is being excreted through the dermis.

Support skin detoxification with regular sweating (sauna, movement), dry brushing, clay masks, sea salt baths, and avoiding petrochemical-based lotions and soaps. What you apply *on* your skin either supports or stresses your inner systems.

Letting the Body Do What is Already Known

The beauty of detox is that the body already knows how. You do not require force. You only create the conditions for the process to happen. Fatigue often begins to lift the moment elimination becomes effortless.

Before supplements, before protocols, and before extreme regimens, the question is simple: *Are the exits open?*

If not, this is the place to begin. When you open the channels, energy returns with grace.

Detox Flow Chart

Open the Exits, Reclaim Your Energy

1. COLON

Signs of Stagnation:

- Constipation
- Bloating
- Brain fog
- Skin breakouts
- Fatigue after meals

How to Restore Flow:

- Hydration
- Raw fruits and leafy greens
- Magnesium (citrate or glycinate)
- Enemas and colonics
- Chia and flaxseed
- Prune or senna tea

2. LIVER

Signs of Stagnation:

- Irritability
- Hormonal imbalance
- Nausea or indigestion
- Fatigue after eating
- Sensitivity to chemicals or fragrances

How to Restore Flow:

- Lemon water on an empty stomach
- Bitter greens (dandelion, arugula)
- Milk thistle and turmeric
- Castor oil packs over the liver
- Light, plant-based eating

3. KIDNEYS

Signs of Stagnation:

- Puffy eyes
- Lower back discomfort
- Dark, strong-smelling urine
- Poor recovery from stress or exercise
- Frequent dehydration

How to Restore Flow:

- Fresh coconut water
- Herbal teas (nettle, parsley, horsetail)
- Watermelon and cucumber
- Structured/mineralized water
- Reduce animal protein and sodium

4. LYMPHATIC SYSTEM

Signs of Stagnation:

- Swollen glands
- Joint stiffness
- Chronic tension or soreness
- Brain fog
- Cellulite or skin eruptions

How to Restore Flow:

- Rebounding or brisk walking
- Dry brushing toward the heart
- Deep breathing
- Lymphatic massage or cupping
- Sauna or cold/hot contrast showers

5. LUNGS

Signs of Stagnation:

- Shallow or rapid breathing
- Anxiety or tight chest
- Poor endurance
- Low oxygen saturation
- Poor sleep quality

How to Restore Flow:

- Diaphragmatic nasal breathing
- Breath holds and rhythmic breathwork
- Air purifiers and open windows
- Avoid synthetic air sprays
- Singing, chanting, or humming

6. SKIN

Signs of Stagnation:

- Acne or rashes
- Body odor
- Dull complexion
- Itching or inflammation

How to Restore Flow:

- Sweat daily (movement or sauna)
- Clay masks and dry brushing
- Sea salt or magnesium baths
- Natural, toxin-free skincare
- Stay well hydrated

Note:

If one detox channel is blocked, others must work harder. The more open the exits, the lighter and more energized your body becomes. Detox is not a crash. This is a return to rhythm.

Chapter 5: Power of the Plant

How Living Foods Reignite Cellular Energy

Fatigue does not thrive in a clean body. Low energy feeds on acids, blockages, residues, and rot that all contribute to stagnation. There is a category of nourishment that speaks directly to the language of life, offering not just calories, but *code*. That nourishment is found in plants. Fresh, living, sun-charged plants. They are not just food. They are frequency. They are the antidote to modern exhaustion.

You were not designed to extract energy from death. Meat, dairy, eggs, and processed animal products burden the lymph, thicken the blood, slow the colon, strain the kidneys, and rot in the gut. These substances are foreign to the electrical intelligence of your body. They may stimulate the system briefly, like fat on a fire, but leave behind the ashes of inflammation, stagnation, and toxicity.

In contrast, plants *cleanse as they nourish.* Their enzymes repair. Their antioxidants disarm free radicals. Their fiber sweeps the intestines. Their water hydrates the cells. Their chlorophyll oxygenates the blood. They work in harmony with your body, not in opposition.

Fruit, especially, is the highest octave of food. This is energy made edible that is solar-powered, alkalizing, hydrating, and electrifying. Fruit requires the least digestive energy while offering the most efficient fuel. Raw fruits and vegetables do not steal your energy to break down, they *give* you energy by how easily they flow through your system.

The Mitochondrial Connection

Your mitochondria thrive on clean glucose, oxygen, minerals, and structured water. These are all abundantly available in whole plant foods. They shut down, however, in the presence of inflammatory compounds, ammonia, uric acid, saturated fats, and metabolic waste. All of which are abundantly found in animal products.

This is not ideology. This is biology. Studies show that saturated fat impairs mitochondrial efficiency and increases free radical production. In contrast, polyphenols, flavonoids, and plant antioxidants *stimulate mitochondrial biogenesis.* The creation of new energy factories inside your cells.

When you eat raw spinach, citrus, berries, sprouts, or drink beet juice, you are not just feeding yourself, you are restoring your cellular engines.

Beets, Blood, and Nitric Oxide

One of the most powerful plant-based energy boosters is *nitric oxide*. This is a gas your body naturally produces to expand blood vessels, improve circulation, and increase oxygen delivery. Few foods support this like beets.

Beet juice has become a performance secret in elite endurance circles. A phenomenon known as *"beet doping."* Rich in dietary nitrates, beets are converted in the mouth and gut into nitric oxide, resulting in increased stamina, lower blood pressure, faster recovery, and more efficient oxygen use at the muscular level.

Citrulline, found in watermelon, also boosts nitric oxide levels, improving blood flow and reducing fatigue. These are not hacks, they are nature's *original design* for endurance, resilience, and flow.

Unlike synthetic energy drinks, which force the body into artificial stimulation and ultimately crash your adrenals, beets and citrulline support the system's *natural rhythm* of circulation and renewal. They do not take, they give.

The Real Cost of Stimulation

Energy drinks, caffeine shots, and pre-workouts are not solutions. They are adrenaline grenades. Most contain synthetic caffeine, artificial sweeteners, dyes, and preservatives that irritate the gut, burden the liver, disrupt the heart, and leave the body more depleted than before.

They do not create energy; they steal tomorrow's vitality to power today's panic. True energy is never frantic. Clean fuel is steady, clean, and quiet in confidence.

Eat to Energize, Not to Escape

Food is either fuel or fog. When you eat in alignment with your design, foods that cleanse, hydrate, remineralize, and move, you become energized not just physically, but mentally, emotionally, and even spiritually. Your thoughts lift. Your breath deepens. Your purpose sharpens. You begin to *feel like yourself again.*

This is what fatigue steals most. The sense of being fully *you*, present, capable, and clear. Let plants be your allies. Not just as food, but as medicine. As memory. As the living keys that unlock your true energy potential.

Top 15 Fatigue-Fighting Plant Foods

The following foods are nature's most potent allies for reversing fatigue, restoring mitochondrial function, and building energy.

1. Beets
Boost nitric oxide for improved oxygen flow and endurance.

2. Watermelon
High in citrulline and hydration, supports kidneys and blood circulation.

3. Blueberries
Packed with antioxidants that protect the brain and mitochondria.

4. Leafy Greens (Spinach, Kale, Dandelion)
Rich in chlorophyll, minerals, & bitter compounds that support the liver.

5. Pineapple
Contains bromelain for digestion and anti-inflammatory support.

6. Avocado
Healthy plant fats, potassium, and magnesium support adrenal function.

7. Lemons
Alkalizing and liver-stimulating; great first thing in the morning.

8. Chia Seeds
Hydrating, fiber-rich, and packed with omega-3s for cellular elasticity.

9. Sprouts (Broccoli, Sunflower, Alfalfa)
Enzyme-rich, living foods that increase vitality and detoxification.

10. Papaya
Digestive enzyme powerhouse with soft, soothing fiber for the gut.

11. Coconut Water
Nature's electrolyte solution. Supports adrenal and kidney health.

12. Sea Moss or Dulse
Provides trace minerals and iodine to support thyroid and energy metabolism.

13. Ginger
Improves digestion, circulation, and lymphatic flow.

14. Cucumber
Hydrating, silica-rich, and excellent for skin and kidney support.

15. Fresh Herbs (Parsley, Cilantro, Basil)
Chelate toxins, improve digestion, and bring life force to meals.

The Daily Energy Plate

Structuring Plant-Based Meals for Mitochondrial Power and Detox Flow

Use this simple framework to build meals that energize rather than exhaust. Each component supports a different aspect of cellular vitality.

1. Raw Hydrating Base (40%)

• Fruit in the morning: papaya, berries, watermelon, mango
• Salads at lunch or dinner: leafy greens, cucumber, sprouts
• Juices or smoothies: green juice, beet-carrot juice, fruit-based smoothies

2. Mineral-Dense Plants (25%)

• Steamed greens: kale, chard, bok choy
• Root veggies: sweet potato, squash, beets
• Cruciferous: broccoli, cauliflower, cabbage

3. Healthy Fats (15%)

• Avocado, flaxseed, chia, hemp, coconut
• Small handful of raw soaked nuts or seeds
• Cold-pressed oils (sparingly): olive or pumpkin seed

4. Clean Proteins (10–15%)

• Lentils, mung beans, chickpeas (well-soaked and cooked)
• Tempeh (soy-free), fermented sprouts, hemp hearts
• Sea vegetables for amino acid variety

5. Functional Add-ons (5%)

• Fresh herbs: parsley, basil, cilantro
• Medicinal spices: turmeric, cinnamon, ginger
• Superfoods: sea moss, spirulina, maca, raw cacao (as needed)

Tip: Always lead your day with fruit or juice, avoid heavy combinations, and honor light digestion. Energy rises when digestion relaxes.

Chapter 6: Fasting & Flow

Reclaiming Energy Through Strategic Emptiness

In a world obsessed with consumption, fasting is a radical act of remembrance. A reminder to the body that energy does not come from constant input, but from intelligent rhythm. Fasting is not starvation. This is *strategic emptiness*. A sacred pause. A biological reset. A way of stepping out of the cycle of fatigue by removing what overwhelms the system.

When the digestive system is constantly processing food, especially heavy or unnatural meals, the body spends a lot of energy breaking down, neutralizing, and eliminating. There is little left for regeneration. When the digestive fire rests, though, that same energy is redirected inward to healing, repair, and renewal.

Fasting liberates the mitochondria, cleans the bloodstream, and awakens autophagy, the body's natural recycling system, which breaks down damaged cells, misfolded proteins, and excess fat stores. In this space of non-eating, your body becomes *metabolically wise*, learning to create energy more efficiently with less.

Far from weakening you, fasting strengthens your adaptability, trains the nervous system to operate in a state of calm clarity without being constantly fueled, and sharpens your mind. Not through stimulation, but through the quiet awakening that happens when you stop distracting yourself with fullness.

Types of Fasting for Fatigue Recovery

Not all fasts are extreme. Not all fasts require deprivation. In fact, the best fasts are gentle, rhythmic, and intentional.

1. Intermittent Fasting
A daily time-restricted eating window (e.g., 8 hours eating, 16 hours fasting) that allows the digestive system to rest and regulate hormones. This is ideal for beginner fasting and daily maintenance.

2. Juice Fasting
A flood of raw, enzymatic hydration that deeply nourishes while freeing the gut from fiber digestion. Green juices, coconut water, and beet-celery-carrot blends can support detox while maintaining energy.

3. Mono Fruit Meals or Fruit-Only Days
Eating one type of fruit per meal, or for a full day, lightens the digestive load, supports lymphatic cleansing, and builds energy without heaviness.

4. Dry Fasting (Advanced)
Short-term fasting with no food or water, done carefully under proper preparation. Dry fasting initiates deep autophagy and tissue cleansing but should be reserved for advanced protocols.

5. Circadian Fasting
Aligning eating windows with natural light cycles. Eating from sunrise to sunset, and nothing after dark. This honors the body's hormonal and digestive clocks.

The Energetics of Emptiness

Fasting opens a quiet space within the body where clarity rushes in. This is energetic, not just physical. Emotional clutter surfaces, mental fog lifts, and fatigue often begins to dissolve. Not because of you adding something, but because you finally allow stillness to work.

In spiritual traditions across the Earth, fasting was used to hear the voice within. To receive guidance. To purify the vessel before prayer. Still today, this remains one of the most effective tools to recalibrate body, mind, and spirit toward vitality.

Signs You May Be Required to Fast

• You feel sluggish after meals.
• Your hunger feels compulsive, not intuitive.
• You wake up tired even after 8+ hours of sleep.
• Your tongue is coated and breath is off.
• You feel "full" even when undernourished.

When done with intention, fasting is reverence, not restriction.

Begin Light. Build Rhythm.

You do not have to start with extremes. Begin with 12–14 hours between dinner and breakfast. Replace one heavy meal with juice. Let your body relearn your rhythm. As you do, your energy will begin to rise. Not in spikes, but in steady waves. True flow, you will realize, comes not just from what you add, but from what you *release.*

Fasting Starter Guide

Begin Gently. Build Rhythm. Activate Energy.

Fasting doesn't need to be extreme to be effective. This guide outlines approachable methods for building a fasting rhythm that restores energy, digestion, and mental clarity—without deprivation.

Beginner Path (Ease-In Strategy)

Goal: Light digestive reset, improved energy awareness.
- Fast 12–14 hours overnight (e.g., 7 PM to 9 AM).
- Eliminate late-night eating.
- Begin each day with warm lemon water or green juice.
- Replace one solid meal with a hydrating smoothie or juice.
- Try one "fruit-only" day per week to lighten the load.

Intermediate Path (Fatigue Recovery Mode)

Goal: Cleanse lymph, enhance mitochondria, improve sleep & focus.
- Fast 14–16 hours overnight (e.g., 6 PM to 10 AM)
- Introduce a weekly 1-day juice fast (vegetable-based)
- Use mono-meals of melon, papaya, or grapes during high-fatigue periods.
- Break fast with enzyme-rich foods (papaya, pineapple, green juice).

Advanced Path (Supervised or Cyclical Use)

Goal: Deep autophagy, cellular recycling, spiritual reset.
- 24-hour liquid fast with herbal teas, water, and juices.
- Dry fasting (no food or water) for 12–18 hours (*only under experience or supervision*).
- Extended juice fasts (3–7 days) with support.
- Align fasting days with rest, nature immersion, and light movement.

Always listen to your body. Fatigue should improve, not worsen, during fasting. Ease is the sign of alignment. Discomfort reveals deeper stagnation.

Daily Fasting Rhythm Template

Structure for Consistent Energy and Digestive Ease

This is a sample 24-hour fasting-friendly rhythm that works for most people seeking gentle detox and stable vitality.

6:30–8:00 AM — Morning Rituals (No Food Yet)
- Hydrate with lemon water or coconut water.
- Gentle movement: walk, breathwork, sunlight.
- Avoid caffeine first 90 minutes.

9:00–10:00 AM — Break Fast Gently
- Option 1: Green juice (celery, cucumber, lemon, apple).
- Option 2: Fruit-only breakfast (papaya, melon, berries).
- Add minerals or herbs if needed (e.g., sea moss, nettle).

12:30–1:30 PM — Light, Alkaline Lunch
- Large raw salad with sprouts, avocado, lemon-olive oil dressing.
- Light steamed vegetables or sweet potato.
- Herbal tea or cucumber-mint water.

3:00–4:00 PM — Midday Reset
- Optional: Small green smoothie or fruit if needed.
- Breathwork, walk, or sunlight break.
- Dry brushing or lymph support practice.

5:30–6:30 PM — Final Meal of the Day
- Steamed vegetables, squash, or millet bowl.
- Warm herbal tea to close digestion.
- No food after 7:00 PM if possible.

8:00–9:00 PM — Evening Wind-Down
- Blue light off, screens dimmed.
- Gratitude journaling or emotional clearing.
- Deep rest by 10:00 PM or earlier.

Consistency builds momentum. Even small fasting windows create space for the body to reset.

Part III: Building Fatigue Immunity

Becoming the Kind of Human That Energy Trusts

There comes a moment, after the detox, after the pause, and after the clearing, when energy begins to return. Not as a spike, or a high, but as a current. Subtle at first, and gentle, like a whisper of strength you almost forgot belonged to you. This is when real transformation begins.

Healing, we discover, is not just about getting rid of what drains you but is about *becoming* someone new. Someone whose body holds energy with grace, whose habits build momentum, and whose choices protect the flame of vitality rather than constantly extinguishing.

Fatigue immunity is not a fantasy. This is a physical *condition*. A pattern of living where your system is no longer overdrawn, overstimulated, or overwhelmed. A way of being where *energy is your default*, not your wish. Attaining this condition is not reserved for the rare or genetically blessed. This is available to anyone willing to live in rhythm, to move with integrity, and to nourish the body as a temple of life.

This next phase of the journey is about cultivation. Learning how to build strength, not through force but through flow. This is about activating muscle, breath, resilience, and joy, and becoming a clear channel. Not just for energy, but for purpose.

You have cleared the static and opened the exits. Now, you begin to *generate*. Now you build energy from the ground up.

Chapter 7: Move to Power

How Vigorous Movement Awakens the Body's Energy Engines

Fatigue often tricks us into stillness, but not the nourishing kind. This pulls us into a paralysis of depletion, where rest becomes avoidance, and movement feels impossible. Yet, paradoxically, the very thing we need to break that cycle is *movement*.

Not frantic exertion, or punishment-driven workouts, but *intentional, rhythmic movement*. The kind that pumps the heart, awakens the lungs, mobilizes the lymph, and whispers to the mitochondria: *This is your time to grow.*

Your body is adaptive, not fragile, and responds to challenge with resilience if that challenge is offered in love. When you move with vitality as your intention, you begin to *build energy, not burn*. This is the forgotten secret of longevity: energy is *generated* by the body in motion.

Mitochondria Love Movement

Every time you engage your muscles, you signal your body to build more mitochondria. This process, called mitochondrial biogenesis, literally *creates more energy-producing factories* inside your cells. The more mitochondria you have, the more oxygen you can use, the more food you can convert to fuel, and the more resilient you become.

Movement activates the lungs, flushes the lymphatic system, massages the organs, oxygenates blood, and strengthens circulation. Being active creates an internal terrain where fatigue cannot thrive.

Not all movements, though, are created equal. The body thrives on variety. Try dynamic bursts, gentle stretches, and rhythmic flow. From barefoot hikes to breath-led yoga, and from rebounding to resistance, every intentional motion becomes a mitochondria love letter. When we move with joy, presence, and breath, we invite vitality to take root. Movement becomes more than exercise. We experience cellular celebration, a daily reminder that energy is not something we chase, but something we cultivate.

The Fatigue-Fighting Movement Trinity

To restore natural energy, you do not need extreme workouts. What you need is consistency, diversity, and intention.

Here is a foundational triad:

1. Vigorous Daily Movement (30–45 min minimum)

- Brisk walking, hiking, rebounding.
- Bodyweight training, functional circuits.
- Dancing, swimming, barefoot running on natural terrain.
- Breath-led movement (Qi Gong, primal flow).

These sessions build strength and lymphatic momentum. The goal is not exhaustion, but *circulation.*

2. Micro-Movement Throughout the Day

- Short walks after meals.
- Stretching breaks every hour.
- Squatting, spinal twists, jumping rope, toe-touches.
- Shake out the limbs, swing the arms, bounce on the heels.

Movement is *medicine*, especially when frequent, not just intensely.

3. Restorative Flow States

- Yoga, slow martial arts, intuitive movement, nature immersion.
- Breath-guided flow to downregulate the nervous system.
- Movement that connects you to pleasure, not performance.

These forms recalibrate the body into harmony, helping integrate strength and stillness.

Lymphatic Liberation

The lymphatic system *depends* on your movement to circulate. There is no pump attached. Without movement, toxins stagnate. With movement, your inner river flows.

Every bounce, stretch, and twist is a signal: *Release. Detox. Reboot.* This is why rebounding (mini trampoline) is one of the most powerful anti-fatigue tools available. Ten minutes a day moves the lymph, strengthens bones, and improves detoxification more efficiently than most supplements.

The Breath-Movement Bridge

Breath is a catalyst, and not just a companion to movement. Syncing breath with motion supercharges the nervous system, deepens oxygen delivery, and activates parasympathetic repair even during vigorous activity.

Try this rhythm during walks or strength sessions:

• **Inhale for 3 steps** → **Hold for 3** → **Exhale for 5** → **Hold for 2.** Repeat. Adjust with your pace. Let this become a moving meditation.

When breath and movement align, the body becomes a prayer in motion. This union calms the mind, focuses intention, and invites flow state. Where effort feels easeful and awareness sharpens. Over time, this practice rewires your response to stress, transforming exertion into empowerment. Here, in the breath-movement bridge, exercise becomes embodied presence rather than punishment, and vitality begins to rise from within.

Move to Feel, Not Just to Fix

This is not about checking boxes. This is about feeling *alive.* Movement reconnects you with your power. The moment the fog lifts, the blood warms, and the spine straightens during exercise is when you stop identifying with fatigue and begin embodying strength again.

So, move, not to chase energy, but to *become the source.* You are not broken. You are simply under-activated. The cure is in your body's favorite language: motion.

Let movement be your remembrance, not your remedy. Dance without reason. Walk without a destination. Stretch because your cells are thirsty for space. When you move to feel, you awaken the joy of being in a body. Not to perfect, but to inhabit with pride. This is how healing begins. Not with a prescription, but with permission to feel yourself fully, again.

Daily Movement Blueprint

Build Energy Through Rhythmic Motion

Use this flexible template to structure your day around energy-generating movement. The goal is consistency, oxygenation, and flow. This rhythm supports detox, circulation, and mitochondrial resilience.

Morning (within 30 minutes of waking):

☐ 5–10 minutes of gentle joint rotations, stretches, or sun salutations.
☐ 5 minutes of breathwork: deep nasal inhales, slow extended exhales.
☐ Optional: light barefoot walk or bounce to awaken lymph.

Midday (11:00 AM–2:00 PM):

☐ 30–45 minutes of vigorous movement (choose one):
  • Brisk walking or hiking.
  • Bodyweight circuit (squats, push-ups, lunges, planks).
  • Rebounding on a mini-trampoline.
  • Dance, martial arts, primal movement flow.
☐ Emphasize nasal breathing and good posture.
☐ Hydrate before and after (coconut water or green juice ideal).

Afternoon Micro-Movement:

☐ 5-minute movement breaks every hour (choose any):
  • Standing forward folds.
  • Deep squats or hip openers.
  • Arm swings, toe touches, spinal twists.
☐ Optional: gentle walk or lymph brushing after lunch.

Evening (Sunset Wind-Down):

☐ 10–20 minutes of restorative movement:
  • Yoga (yin, gentle flow, or restorative).
  • Qi Gong or tai chi-style breath-led movements.
  • Grounding (walk in nature, barefoot if possible).
☐ Close with 3–5 minutes of stillness or box breathing (4-4-4-4 rhythm).

Note: Movement does not deplete you when done *for energy, not ego*. Listen to your body. Feel your breath. Let joy guide the way.

Lymphatic Activation Routine

Flush Stagnation. Restore Flow. Support Detox.

The lymphatic system is your body's internal drainage network. Optimal lymph flow requires your participation. This simple routine, done daily or as needed, helps reduce inflammation, support immunity, and release fatigue.

Duration: 10–20 minutes.

Frequency: 1–2x per day (especially in the morning).

1. Dry Brushing (2–5 minutes):

- Use a natural bristle brush on dry skin.
- Always brush *toward the heart.*
- Start at feet and work upward: legs, abdomen, arms, chest.
- Light, sweeping strokes. Avoid face and broken skin.

2. Rebounding or Bouncing (5–10 minutes):

- Jump on a mini-trampoline or bounce gently on the balls of your feet
- Keep arms loose and jaw relaxed
- If no trampoline: bounce in place, shake limbs, or do jumping jacks
- Breathe deep through your nose while moving

3. Breathwork Booster (3–5 minutes):

Try this lymph-clearing pattern:

- Inhale (4 seconds) → Hold (4) → Exhale (6–8) → Pause (2).
- Repeat 10–15 rounds.
- Optional: Add humming on the exhale to vibrate lymph-rich throat.

4. Contrast Shower (Optional, 3–5 minutes):

- Alternate 30 seconds hot / 30 seconds cold water for 4–6 rounds.
- Always end with cold.
- Rub skin vigorously with a towel afterward to stimulate flow.

Quick Add-Ons:

☐ Walk briskly for 20 minutes.

☐ Lay flat with legs up the wall for 5–10 minutes.

☐ Sip warm lemon water or herbal lymph tea (red clover, burdock).

If you feel foggy, puffy, or stuck, move your lymph. Energy follows circulation. Freedom begins in flow.

Chapter 8: Sleep Like a Sage

Restoring Energy Through Deep, Rhythmic Sleep

Fatigue cannot be healed without sleep. You can cleanse your organs, eat the cleanest food, and move with perfect rhythm but if your sleep is shallow, fragmented, or misaligned with nature, your body will remain in deficit. Sleep is not a passive state; this is active repair. A sacred recalibration. The time when your brain detoxifies, tissues regenerate, immune system reboots, and hormones reset. In a world of screens, stress, stimulants, and artificial light, however, true sleep has become rare. Most people are *unconscious* at night but very few are actually *rested*.

To sleep like a sage is to restore a sacred rhythm. This means honoring your circadian clock, preparing the body for nightfall, and entering sleep with the reverence of a ritual. Not collapsing from exhaustion but entering rest *intentionally*.

The sage does not chase sleep; he creates the conditions for sleep to arrive. Cool darkness, slow breath, and a nervous system softened by stillness. Screens are set aside, meals are digested, thoughts are cleared like ashes from a hearth. Melatonin rises when light recedes. Growth hormone pulses when the body surrenders. Deep sleep is not just recovery but is remembering. This is the nightly return to the origin of self, where healing is not forced but invited through rhythm, quiet, and care.

The Physiology of Restoration

During deep sleep (especially stages N3 and REM), your glymphatic system flushes waste from your brain, clearing amyloid plaques and neurotoxins. Your liver regenerates. Growth hormone surges. Muscle fibers repair. Cortisol drops. Melatonin rises. Your immune system scans pathogens and resets inflammation.

While the lymphatic system clears waste from the body, the glymphatic system is the brain's unique cleansing network that operates primarily during deep sleep, flushing out cellular debris, toxins, and metabolic waste through cerebrospinal fluid. Unlike the rest of the body's lymphatic vessels, the glymphatic system flows along glial cells. Hence the name *"glymphatic."* This is a nightly rinse cycle for the brain, clearing out what could contribute to brain fog, neurodegeneration, or fatigue. Movement, hydration, and quality sleep all support both systems, because when drainage flows, energy follows.

Why Most People Sleep Poorly

When rhythms are disrupted, no amount of supplements or smoothies can replace what sleep alone is designed to do. Sleep was once effortless. Cradled by moonlight, cooled by earth, and synced with the rising and setting of the sun. In the modern world, though, we have forgotten how to fall into rest. Our biology has not changed, but our environments, habits, and thoughts have. We have created a culture that glorifies productivity and neglects recovery, pushing the body into chronic overdrive while starving for repair.

Sleep is nature's original medicine, but modern life has made us resistant to the embrace. We have traded campfires for screens, stillness for scrolling, and rest for artificial stimulation. The result? A generation tired but wired, craving energy but sabotaging the rhythms that restore.

These are some reasons why many people sleep poorly:

• Overexposure to blue light and screens at night.

• Stimulants (coffee, sugar, energy drinks) late in the day.

• Eating late or consuming heavy meals before bed.

• Elevated cortisol from stress and unresolved emotions.

• Disconnection from natural light cycles and daily movement.

•Sleeping in EMF-heavy environments.

• Excessive exposure to indoor lighting after sunset, disrupting melatonin production.

• Mental overstimulation from late-night work, social media, or emotional conflict.

• Lack of mineral-rich hydration, leading to cramping or restless sleep.

• Shallow breathing patterns and poor CO_2 tolerance inhibiting nervous system downregulation.

• Overheating the bedroom or sleeping in synthetic, non-breathable bedding.

Modern sleep is distorted, not just insufficient. We go to bed overstimulated, undergrounded, and emotionally unprocessed. In doing so, we rob the body of a nightly healing window. True rest begins with remembering we are animals of rhythm. When we rise with the light, move with the day, and dim with the dusk, sleep no longer needs to be chased but returns like a faithful tide.

Reclaiming the Rhythm

The goal is not just more sleep, but *better sleep*. Here is how to restore the deep, rhythmic cycles your body craves:

1. Honor the Sunset
• Dim your lights after dusk.
• Avoid screens or use blue-light filters.
• Light candles, read printed books, or play calming music.
• Let your body *know* that night has arrived.

2. Establish a Sleep Ritual
• Herbal tea (chamomile, skullcap, passionflower or Spring Dragon).
• Gentle yoga or breathwork (e.g., 4-7-8 pattern).
• Journaling to clear emotional residue.
• Magnesium bath or castor oil foot rub.
• Consistent bedtime (ideally by 10:00 PM).

3. Create a Sacred Sleep Space
• Remove electronics and Wi-Fi sources.
• Keep the room cool, dark, and quiet.
• Use blackout curtains and a grounding sheet if possible.
• Sleep on natural materials (cotton, linen, organic bedding).
• Keep phones out of the room or on airplane mode.

4. Align With the Earth
• Get sunlight in your eyes within thirty minutes of waking.
• Walk barefoot on natural ground to reset circadian rhythm.
• Open windows or spend time outdoors daily.
• Connect with the seasons. Eat, move, and rest accordingly.
• Let nature, not algorithms, set your internal clock.

5. Prepare the Mind for Stillness
• Avoid stimulating conversations or content before bed.
• Practice gratitude or prayer to shift from thinking to feeling.
• Release unresolved thoughts through "mental dumping" on paper.
• Try binaural beats or delta wave soundscapes.
• Enter sleep like a ceremony. Not as escape, but as return.

Rewriting Your Sleep Identity

Many people unknowingly identify with being a *"light sleeper," "night owl,"* or *"insomniac."* These labels become self-fulfilling prophecies. Your biology is ancient, though. You are wired for sleep. What is required is not to *force* sleep, but to *remove what disrupts*, and to build trust in your body's rhythm again.

Your sleep story can change. Identity is elastic and is shaped by repetition, not destiny. Each time you choose to dim the lights, to breathe deeply, or to lie down with presence rather than pressure, you are rewriting the script. You are teaching your nervous system safety, not struggle. Over time, the story of *"I do not sleep well"* is replaced by *"I know how to rest."* This is not about perfection, but pattern. Every night is a chance to begin again.

Daytime Determines Nighttime

How you move, eat, breathe, and focus during the day determines how deeply you rest at night. Morning sunlight, movement, and mineral-rich foods signal the clock. Avoiding stimulants after noon and finishing your last meal early tell the body, *"We are safe. We can rest."*

Rest is not something that begins at bedtime. You build this all day long. Each moment of presence, each deep breath, and each aligned choice nourishes the rhythm that leads you into sleep. When you ground your body to the Earth, hydrate with intention, and pause between tasks, you are telling your nervous system not to stay on guard. Evening sleep is earned not through exhaustion, but through a day lived in coherence.

Sleep Is Leadership, not Laziness

To reclaim your energy, you must reclaim your sleep. Not just in quantity but in quality, rhythm, and intention. In a culture that glorifies hustle and caffeine, choosing to sleep like a sage is an act of rebellion. A return to wisdom.

Those who rest well lead well. Sleep sharpens intuition, regulates emotion, strengthens immunity, and restores clarity. This is the foundation beneath every inspired decision, and every courageous act. To prioritize sleep is not to slow down but to rise rooted. In honoring rest, you model a new paradigm: one where power is sourced from alignment, not adrenaline.

Sleep Optimization Checklist

Clear the Interference. Let Sleep Do Its Work.

Use this checklist to support deep, regenerative sleep. Even a few changes can dramatically improve your nighttime recovery and next-day energy.

Sleep Environment

☐ Remove all electronic devices (or place on airplane mode).
☐ Shut off Wi-Fi router at night.
☐ Use blackout curtains or eye mask to block all light.
☐ Keep room cool (60–67°F / 15–19°C ideal).
☐ Invest in natural fiber bedding and breathable sheets.
☐ Eliminate synthetic scents (no dryer sheets, plug-ins, or candles).

Evening Nutrition & Rhythm

☐ Eat your last meal at least 3 hours before bed
☐ Avoid caffeine after 12:00 PM
☐ Limit alcohol and processed sugars
☐ Drink herbal tea (e.g., chamomile, lemon balm, skullcap)
☐ Consider magnesium glycinate or topical magnesium oil

Light & Circadian Support

☐ Get 10–20 minutes of natural light before 10:00 AM
☐ Dim indoor lighting after sunset
☐ Avoid screens 1 hour before bed (or use blue-light blockers)
☐ Use candles, salt lamps, or red lights in the evening

Body & Mind Preparation

☐ Do gentle movement or breathwork (4-7-8 or box breathing)
☐ Journal or reflect to process thoughts/emotions
☐ Try warm baths, castor oil packs, or foot soaks
☐ Use a calming nighttime affirmation or visualization

Sleep is not a luxury. This is your foundation. Build a sanctuary around the importance of adequate rest, and your energy will rise naturally.

Evening Wind-Down Routine Template

Signal the Body. Soften the Mind. Prepare for Deep Rest.

Use or customize the flow below to create your personalized pre-sleep ritual. The goal is *consistency and ease,* repeating calming signals that invite parasympathetic repair.

2–3 Hours Before Bed

- Finish the last meal (light, plant-based preferred).
- Dim lights or switch to red/orange tones.
- Turn off screens or wear blue-light blocking glasses.
- Light candles, incense, or use warm-toned lighting.

1 Hour Before Bed

- Make herbal tea (chamomile, passionflower, reishi, or valerian root).
- Take a warm shower, Epsom salt bath, or use magnesium spray.
- Practice gentle stretching or yoga.
- Write down thoughts, to-dos, or a gratitude list in a journal.

15–30 Minutes Before Bed

- Do breathwork: 4-7-8 or slow nasal breathing (5–10 rounds).
- Read a printed book or spiritual passage (avoid screens).
- Optional: foot massage with castor oil or calming balm.
- Lay in bed with no stimulation. Use darkness as medicine.

Bedtime Intention (Optional):

Say aloud or inwardly: *"I release today. I invite deep rest. I allow healing to unfold as I sleep."*

Chapter 9: The Anti-Fatigue Lifestyle

Living in Rhythm with Vitality

Energy is something you cultivate, not chase. Once you have cleared the burdens, opened the exits, nourished your cells, and reclaimed your rest, the final step is to *design your life around energy*. Not just avoiding what depletes you but choosing what fuels you every day.

This is the anti-fatigue lifestyle: a pattern of living that protects your vitality, honors your rhythms, and reinforces everything you have rebuilt. This is not about restriction but perfection. Making choices that match the truth of who you are and how your body was designed to thrive.

The New Way of Being

This lifestyle is not built on hacks or discipline alone. This way of life is constructed on *knowing*. The felt sense of how to live with clarity in your breath, softness in your belly, and electricity in your bones. You do not need to do everything. You only need to do what matters, *reliably.*

Vitality is a frequency, not a finish line. The more often you tune in, the more naturally you elevate. You notice how your body speaks: through cravings, through tension, and through joy. You start to design your days like a garden, protecting your mornings, pruning your inputs, and planting recovery between exertion. The anti-fatigue lifestyle is about rhythm, not intensity. Rhythm is what turns habits into harmony.

You are not here to survive your days. You are here to create them. When you live in sync with your biology and protect your energy like sacred currency, fatigue no longer has a foothold. What emerges instead is a new way of being that is rooted, radiant, and ready. Not because life has got easier, but because *you* became aligned.

Morning: Momentum with Meaning

Mornings set the tone for the entire nervous system. When you wake *with intention*, you shift from reaction to creation.

Anti-Fatigue Morning Essentials:

- Rise with natural light or sunlight within thirty minutes.
- Hydrate immediately: lemon water, juice, or structured water.
- Move your body: walk, bounce, stretch, sunbathe, squat.
- Breathe with presence (5–10 minutes of breathwork or silence).
- Eat a clean, hydrating breakfast (fruit, green juice, smoothie).
- Avoid screens, caffeine, and conflict during the first hour.

Start your day from overflow, not survival.

Midday: Energy Preservation and Alignment

Afternoons are when many people hit their energetic low. With the right practices, this becomes a zone of expansion, not collapse.

Midday Anchors:

- Eat a raw-based lunch (greens, fruits, sprouts, healthy fats).
- Take a short post-meal walk for digestion and lymph flow.
- Avoid stimulants, heavy grains, or processed snacks.
- Block time for focused work and breathing room.
- Touch nature, feel your body, and move every hour.

Fatigue often returns when you forget to feel your body. Reconnect regularly.

Evening: Transition, Not Shutdown

Evenings are not a time to *crash*; they are a time to *decelerate*. This is when your body prepares for deep repair.

Anti-Fatigue Evening Rituals:

- Finish eating by 6:30–7:00 PM if possible.
- Dim lights and reduce screen exposure after sunset.
- Take a walk or do light movement to release tension.
- Use journaling, herbal tea, magnesium, or breath to unwind.
- Enter sleep as a ceremony, not as an escape.

Guarding Your Energy Environment

Your lifestyle is not just made of routines. This is made of environments, relationships, and inputs. Protect what supports your vitality.

Environmental Fatigue Triggers to Minimize:

• EMFs (turn off Wi-Fi at night, avoid sleeping with phones).
• Synthetic chemicals (cleaners, fragrances, water contaminants).
• Excess noise, light pollution, and mental overstimulation.
• Emotional drains: unresolved conflict, boundary breaches, and negative news cycles.

Build a Sanctuary Life by Adding:

• Plants, air purifiers, sunlight, and grounded surfaces.
• Daily nature exposure (forest, beach, sun, soil, stars).
• Music that soothes and uplifts.
• Relationships that honor your energy, not require your depletion.

Fatigue Immunity Is a Lifestyle Choice

You are not fragile; you are programmable. The way you live, your food, movement, breath, thoughts, sleep, and emotional hygiene, becomes the foundation of your energetic reality.

When energy becomes your priority, everything else becomes easier. As your energy rises, so does your ability to create, serve, love, and *remember who you are.*

Anti-Fatigue Daily Tracker

Use this tracker daily or weekly to help build consistency, identify energy patterns, and stay aligned with your anti-fatigue lifestyle.

Morning Energy Rituals

☐ Woke with or near sunrise.
☐ Hydrated before caffeine or food.
☐ Got natural sunlight within 30 min.
☐ Movement (walk, bounce, stretch, breathwork).
☐ Nourished with fruit, green juice, or smoothie.
☐ Avoided screens and stimulation first hour.

Midday Anchors

☐ Plant-based, clean, raw-forward lunch.
☐ Movement after eating (walk or bounce).
☐ Deep breaths or mini-breaks every hour.
☐ No caffeine or sugar crashes.
☐ Time in nature (or grounded setting).

Evening Wind-Down

☐ Finished eating by 7:00 PM.
☐ Dimmed lights and cut screen exposure.
☐ Relaxing movement or emotional clearing.
☐ Magnesium, herbal tea, or grounding.
☐ Asleep by 10:00 PM.

Bonus Practices

☐ Dry brushing, sauna, or lymph support.
☐ Rebounding or cardio session (30–45 min).
☐ Intentional journaling or meditation.

How Was Your Energy Today?

☐ Clear & strong.
☐ Spiky but functional.
☐ Drained & foggy.
☐ Burnt out.

What Helped Most Today?
What Drained You Today?

The 7 Pillars of the Fatigue-Free Life

A Quick Reference Guide to Sustainable Energy

Each of these pillars supports your body's natural energy system. Strengthen these daily, and fatigue will fade from identity to memory.

1. Purification

Clear the internal burden. Open detox channels. Remove toxins, stagnation, and energetic debris.

2. Plant Power

Fuel the body with clean, living food. Hydrate, alkalize, and mineralize with nature's most vibrant medicine.

3. Restorative Sleep

Honor circadian rhythm. Create sacred sleep rituals. Deep rest rebuilds everything.

4. Strategic Fasting

Use emptiness as a healing tool. Allow digestion to rest and energy to reallocate.

5. Rhythmic Movement

Move with intention. Build mitochondrial density. Let the body flow, breathe, sweat, and reset.

6. Nervous System Regulation

Shift from fight-or-flight to rest-and-digest. Breathe deeply. Slow down. Create internal safety.

7. Environmental Harmony

Live in alignment with nature. Minimize EMFs, synthetic chemicals, and overstimulation. Surround yourself with peace.

Fatigue is not who you are. Vitality is your birthright. Build your life around these pillars, and energy will become your new baseline.

Chapter 10: The Breath–Movement Bridge

Synchronizing Breath and Motion for Limitless Energy

The Forgotten Connection

Breath is the conductor of our entire performance. Every step, lift, twist, and bend you take is either powered by oxygen or hindered by an absence of. Yet, most people move with breath as an afterthought, falling into shallow, erratic patterns that keep the nervous system in a state of low-grade stress.

When breath and movement are brought into harmony, a new kind of energy emerges. Not the erratic surge you get from caffeine or adrenaline, but a steady, renewable current that supports endurance, power, recovery, and mental clarity. This is the Breath–Movement Bridge, and when constructed efficiently, fatigue begins to dissolve at the roots.

The bridge is built with a combination of awareness and effort. When you notice how each inhale steadies your spine and every exhale anchors your muscles, movement transforms from something mechanical into being rhythmic. The breath becomes the silent partner in every action, ensuring that energy is released in precise amounts rather than wasted in shallow bursts. This is why elite athletes, martial artists, and yogis all emphasize breathing technique as much as form, because without conscious breath, form eventually collapses.

Modern science validates what ancient wisdom has always taught: oxygen is more than fuel; this is also a catalyst for information. The depth and pace of your breath signal to your nervous system whether you are safe, under threat, or in balance. Shallow, chaotic breathing tells the body to conserve energy in panic, while steady, synchronized breathing communicates that the body can release energy with confidence. This explains why controlled breathing not only enhances physical stamina but also sharpens focus, stabilizes emotions, and prevents burnout.

Think of the Breath–Movement Bridge as an internal technology. A built-in system designed to conserve life force. Once you learn to cross this bridge, every workout, every walk, and even every chore can become a practice in energy efficiency. Instead of draining vitality with unconscious motion, you replenish with deliberate breath. Over time, this does not just improve performance; this rewires the body to resist fatigue, reminding you that vitality is less about pushing harder and more about aligning breath with the natural flow of movement.

Why Breath Synchronization Works

1. Nervous System Reset

Your breathing pattern is a direct switch for your autonomic nervous system. Fast, shallow breathing signals stress. Slow, rhythmic breathing signals safety. When you link intentional breath to movement, you condition your nervous system to stay calm and coherent even under physical demand.

2. Oxygen Efficiency

Not just how much oxygen you inhale but how well your cells utilize oxygen. Intentional breathing improves oxygen delivery to muscles and prevents the buildup of waste products like lactic acid, reducing post-exercise soreness and fatigue.

3. CO_2 Tolerance and Energy

Most fatigue during exertion comes not from lack of oxygen but from the body's intolerance to rising CO_2 levels. Training breath during movement increases CO_2 tolerance, which means you can work harder and longer without feeling *"winded."*

4. Core Stability

Breath integrates with the diaphragm to stabilize the spine, engage deep abdominal muscles, and prevent energy leaks through poor posture or injury.

5. Mental Clarity

Breath-paced movement draws you into a moving meditation. Perceived effort decreases, focus sharpens, and exercise becomes a state of flow rather than strain.

Ancient & Cultural Roots

Breath–movement practices are more than performance enhancers. They are fatigue antidotes woven into culture. Across civilizations, the merging of respiration and rhythm was seen as medicine: to steady the heart, to focus the mind, and to preserve strength for life's demands. Modern science now confirms what these ancient practitioners intuited, that synchronized breathing optimizes oxygen delivery, balances the nervous system, and reduces metabolic stress.

When breath leads our movement, the body expends less energy while producing more power, resilience, and clarity. In this way, these timeless traditions illuminate a truth that speaks directly to our era of exhaustion: *fatigue is not overcome by pushing harder, but by remembering how to breathe in harmony with motion.*

Breath–movement integration is not new. Ancient traditions understood this connection long before modern exercise science:

- **Pranayama & Yoga:** Indian yogis developed breath ratios to guide every posture, believing that breath controls life force (*prana*).

- **Tai Chi & Qi Gong:** Chinese martial artists synchronized breath with slow, precise movements to balance energy flow (*qi*) and longevity.

- **Greek Athletes:** Ancient Olympians trained in breath pacing to improve endurance during running and wrestling.

- **Freedivers:** Modern freedivers condition their breath to conserve oxygen and extend physical capacity far beyond the average person's comfort zone.

These traditions all teach one truth: movement without conscious breath is incomplete.

The 3–Step Breath–Movement Formula

Step 1: Anchor the Rhythm

Choose a breath pattern that matches your activity. For walking, this may be inhaling for three steps, then exhaling for five. For strength training, inhale during lowering, exhale during exertion.

Step 2: Match the Effort

- Endurance → longer exhales for efficiency.
- Steady pace → equal inhale and exhale.
- Short bursts → forceful exhales for power.

Step 3: Stay Present

Let each inhale be a reset and each exhale be a release. Your attention stays on breath as your body's metronome.

When you combine these steps, breath transforms from an unconscious reflex into a performance tool. Anchoring rhythm, matching effort, and staying present form a cycle that prevents wasted energy. Instead of slipping into shallow, erratic breathing that drains stamina, you create an oxygen economy. Each inhale fuels tissues efficiently, while every exhale removes fatigue-causing waste gases. Over time, this practice trains the nervous system to remain calm under stress and teaches the muscles to work with less strain.

This formula also acts as a safeguard against mental exhaustion. Breath is a portable anchor that keeps awareness in the present moment, cutting through distraction and anxiety that deplete energy even faster than physical exertion. Whether in a gym, on a trail, or moving through daily tasks, the purifier's breath–movement formula becomes a way of conserving life force. This transforms ordinary activity into a resilience practice. One that steadily builds endurance not just in the body, but in mind and spirit as well.

Practice Routines

1. Breath–Movement Meditation Walk

- Inhale for three steps → Hold for two steps → Exhale for five steps → Hold for one step.
- Begin with five minutes, progress to twenty.
- Focus on soft, quiet footfalls and nasal breathing.

2. Strength Training Breath

- **Exertion Phase (push/pull/lift):** Exhale fully.
- **Lowering/Returning Phase:** Inhale fully to prepare.
- This stabilizes the core and prevents pressure spikes.

3. Flexibility & Flow

- Inhale with opening/lengthening movements.
- Exhale with closing/folding/twisting movements.
- Keep breath slow to prevent overstretching.

4. Morning Energizer

- Three minutes of gentle bouncing or shaking with deep nasal breathing.
- Inhale through the nose for four counts, exhale through the mouth for six.
- Finish with one minute of stillness.

5. Evening Wind-Down

- Gentle stretching with a four-second inhale, seven-second hold, and eight-second exhale.
- Signals the parasympathetic system to prepare for rest.

Common Mistakes & Fixes

- **Breath-Holding Without Awareness:** Only use the Valsalva maneuver intentionally for max lifts, never for casual reps.
- **Over-Breathing:** Too much oxygen in, not enough CO_2 retained. This leads to dizziness and fatigue. Slow down.
- **Mouth Breathing by Default:** Nasal breathing filters, humidifies, and regulates airflow. Reserve mouth breathing for high intensity bursts.

Case Study: From Winded to Winning

A client named Daniel struggled to run more than two miles without stopping. By incorporating a 3–3 breath pattern (inhale three steps, exhale three steps) and nasal breathing, his endurance doubled in six weeks. He reported feeling less anxious, more present, and recovered faster. This was not because he trained harder, but because he trained smarter through the Breath–Movement Bridge.

Self-Testing & Tools

- **CO_2 Tolerance Test:** Sit, exhale gently, hold breath, and time until first strong urge to inhale. Improving this number improves endurance.
- **Metronome Breathing:** Use a metronome or app to keep breath cadence during movement.
- **Integration in Daily Life:** Apply breath pacing to climbing stairs, carrying groceries or even standing from a chair.

The Anti-Fatigue Edge

When you integrate breath with movement, you stop operating in bursts and crashes. Instead, you build an internal current that is steady, renewable, and deeply reliable. Your body learns to perform in balance, and your mitochondria starts to trust your rhythm. Breath becomes your bridge, and on the other side is a kind of energy you no longer must chase.

Part IV: The Integration of Vitality

Emotional, Purposeful, and Environmental Energy

Energy is not only a matter of mitochondria and movement. This is also the weight of what we carry, the truth we embody, and the environments that surround us. Fatigue is emotional, spiritual, and ecological, in addition to being physical.

This part is about integration. Bringing together the inner and outer worlds. Clearing not only the toxins in the body but also the unspoken words, the unlived purposes, and the unseen environmental drains.

Here, vitality becomes whole. Not a practice you visit, but a way of living. A current that runs through feeling, meaning, and place. This is steady, renewable, and deeply human.

To live without fatigue is not merely to restore the body, but to realign the soul. When your emotions flow freely, your purpose is alive, and your environment is designed to support you, energy becomes a natural state rather than a fleeting experience. This is the point where health and wholeness merge into the same river.

Integration is the art of coherence. Every choice, breath, and space reflect the same truth. When you live this way, energy is no longer chased or borrowed. Vitality becomes the ground you walk on, the rhythm you move with, and the presence you offer to the world.

Chapter 11: Emotional Energy Leaks

The Hidden Drain of Unfelt Feelings

Fatigue is not always physical. Often, you are simply experiencing the weight of what has not been spoken, the grief that has not been cried, and the tension that has been worn like armor for years. Sometimes, you are not tired because you have done too much, but because you have held too much inside.

The body remembers what the mind avoids. Each time you suppress a feeling, deny what is true, or override your emotional needs, the nervous system pays the cost. Not in drama but in depletion. Your energy leaks quietly, and invisibly, into the unexpressed corners of your inner world.

The High Cost of Holding Things Together

Many of us were taught to *"be strong," "stay calm," "get over it,"* or *"keep going."* While these phrases may sound noble, they often become walls that keep our pain locked in. What the body represses must eventually be expressed and we often experience this through chronic tension, digestive issues, shallow breathing, tight fascia, or the constant low hum of fatigue.

Every unprocessed emotion becomes a debt the body must carry. Anger swallowed. Sadness masked. Joy withheld. All of this becomes weight. You begin to feel tired for no apparent reason, because your energy is being used not to *live*, but to *contain*.

Common Emotional Energy Leaks

• Saying *"yes"* when you mean *"no"*.
• People-pleasing or shapeshifting to be accepted.
• Replaying the past or projecting into the future.
• Suppressing anger, grief, or fear.
• Staying silent when your expression needs to be voiced.
• Fearing judgment for your authenticity.
• Betraying your values to keep the peace.

Each of these is a leak. Not always dramatic but deeply draining. When they accumulate, the soul begins to whisper, *"I am tired of not being myself."*

The Nervous System and Truth

When you live in emotional honesty, your body relaxes. The breath deepens. The jaw softens. The immune system is restored. The parasympathetic nervous system comes online. Not because of a pill or supplement, but because you have chosen *congruence.*

There is nothing more regulating to the nervous system than to tell the truth. Not the performative truth. Not the curated version. But the raw, messy, heart-centered truth that says, *"This is what I feel. This is what I need. This is who I am."*

When truth is withheld, the body pays the price. Suppressed feelings tighten muscles, accelerate the pulse, and keep cortisol dripping into the bloodstream like a slow poison. Over time, this constant inner conflict mimics the very stress responses we are trying to escape, draining vitality and clouding clarity. By contrast, honesty unclenches the body's fist. It signals safety at the deepest level, telling the nervous system it no longer needs to guard against its own owner. In this way, truth is not only moral medicine but biological medicine — a detox for the psyche that reverberates through every cell.

Feeling Is Flow

Emotions are not problems. They are portals. When felt fully, without resistance, they pass through. When blocked, they fester. To restore energy, we must restore *permission* to feel, to cry, to rage, to laugh, to tremble, and to release. Feeling is *fluidity,* not weakness. Energy returns when you stop trying to hold everything in place.

Every emotion carries momentum, like a wave that rises to crest and then dissolves. When you allow yourself to ride that wave, it completes its cycle and leaves you lighter than before. But when you dam the current — by suppressing tears, silencing anger, or numbing fear — the water turns stagnant, draining vitality and breeding exhaustion. Feeling is not indulgence; it is hygiene. It keeps the inner rivers clear so that energy can circulate freely, leaving the nervous system resilient and the body unburdened.

Practices to Seal the Leaks

1. Emotional Honesty Inventory

Take time each day or week to ask:
• What am I not saying?
• What am I pretending is fine but is not?
• Where am I shrinking or performing?

2. Embodied Release

• Let yourself cry fully.
• Scream into a pillow or while driving.
• Shake, dance, punch a cushion.
• Write letters you do not send.

3. Speak Your Truth (Safely)
• Practice saying how you feel even if your voice trembles.
• Name your needs without apology.
• Say "no" without explanation.
• Say "yes" without guilt.

4. Breathe Into the Body

• Use breath to explore tight spaces: jaw, chest, belly.
• Ask the tension: "What are you holding?"
• Stay present and allow yourself to speak.

5. Ground Through Nature

• Place bare feet on soil, sand, or stone.
• Imagine excess tension draining down into the earth.
• Let the ground hold what you no longer need to carry.
• Use water (river, ocean, shower) as a ritual of release, letting it wash away residue.

6. Ritual of Reflection

• Set aside a few minutes at day's end to journal honestly about what felt heavy, what felt true, and what you left unspoken.
• Burn or bury pages you don't want to keep, symbolically releasing them.
• Close with one gratitude, reminding the nervous system it is safe to rest.

The Return of Energy

As the emotional body unfreezes, energy begins to return. This does not happen in spikes, but in wholeness. This is not just about having more energy but about no longer wasting the energy you already have. You do not need to be emotionally perfect. You just need to be emotionally honest. The soul does not get tired from doing too much but from not being expressed.

When the backlog of unspoken truths, suppressed grief, and silenced desires begins to move, the body no longer needs to keep the gates locked. Vitality flows differently, in a steady, sustainable, and rooted way. You stop living in reaction and start living in creation. In that shift, fatigue becomes less about depletion and more about misalignment. Something you can address, rather than endure.

This is the kind of energy that does not need caffeine, adrenaline, or crisis to stay active. This is generated from coherence. Your thoughts, emotions, and actions moving in the same direction. When life inevitably brings challenge, this energy does not vanish. We learn to bend without breaking, adapt without abandoning our identity, and become a quiet power we can trust.

Energy born from honesty is self-reinforcing. Each time you speak truth, release grief, or honor desire, you signal to the body to relax from vigilance. Muscles unclench, digestion improves, breath deepens, and the immune system stands down from constant alert. What was once drained in inner conflict is now freed for expansion of creativity, focus, and joy. Over time, this reclaimed current of vitality becomes more reliable than any external stimulant because this is fostered from internal alignment rather than from adrenaline.

This return of energy also changes how you relate to the world. Instead of being tossed by every demand or depleted by every encounter, you carry an inner reserve that makes you less reactive and more intentional. Challenges are still present, but they no longer define your baseline. You become the kind of person who restores quickly, who meets difficulty without collapsing, and who radiates a steadiness that others can feel. This is durable clarity. The kind that turns fatigue into fuel for deeper resilience.

Seal the Leaks: Journal Prompts for Emotional Clarity

Release the Hidden Drains. Reclaim Your Truth.

Use these prompts as daily or weekly practice to explore where your energy may be leaking emotionally. Be honest. Be gentle. Let the page become your clearing ground.

1. Where am I saying "yes" when I mean "no"?

• How would I feel if I were to honor my real answer?

2. Where in my life am I holding something in?

• What truth have I been afraid to speak?

3. What emotion have I been avoiding or suppressing?

• If I let this surface, what might I feel?

4. Who or what drains me consistently and why do I allow this?

• What boundary needs to be placed or reinforced?

5. What part of myself am I afraid to fully express?

• What am I protecting by staying small?

6. What am I grieving, but have not given time or space to feel?

• Can I create a ritual of release?

7. What would I do or say today if I were fully honest?

• Where in my body do I feel that truth living?

Your fatigue may not be a flaw. This may be your soul's way of saying: "Let me speak."

Somatic Release Toolkit

Move Emotion. Free the Body. Return to Flow.

The body holds what the mind suppresses. Use these practices to safely move emotion through the body so that energy can flow again. Start slow. Let sensation, not story, guide the release.

1. Shake Out (2–5 minutes)

• Stand with feet wide, knees soft.
• Begin shaking your hands, then arms, then legs.
• Let your jaw loosen, eyes blink, breath move freely.
• Make sounds if they want to emerge.
• Allow chaos. This is cellular unfreezing.

2. Vocal Release (1–3 minutes)

• In private, scream into a pillow or in the car.
• Use guttural tones, wails, or growls. No censoring.
• Breathe deeply before and after.
• Follow with gentle humming or singing to soothe.

3. Breath & Pressure Point Reset (3–5 minutes)

• Lie down and place one hand on your chest, one on your belly.
• Inhale slowly through your nose for four seconds.
• Exhale audibly through the mouth for six to eight seconds.
• With each exhale, soften a part of your body holding tension.
• Optional: press into the solar plexus or jaw with light touch.

4. Movement Alchemy (5–10 minutes)

• Put on music that evokes what you need to release.
• Let your body move by stomping, curling, shaking, or reaching.
• No choreography. No rules. Just release.
• End in stillness. Let silence be the integration.

5. Grief Ritual (as needed)

• Light a candle.
• Speak aloud who or what you are grieving.
• Let tears come without apology.
• Breathe into your heart or place a hand over.
• When you are ready, blow out the candle as a symbol of release.

Chapter 12: Purpose as Fuel

Why Soul Alignment Restores Energy

You can detox your organs, nourish your mitochondria, and master your sleep but if you are living a life that feels meaningless, misaligned, or muted, fatigue will return. Not because your body is failing but because your *spirit is whispering*, and you are not listening.

Fatigue is existential. The slow erosion of energy that happens when your daily actions betray your deeper knowing. When you work jobs that numb you, speak words that are not true, perform roles that are not yours, or suppress the callings that keep resurfacing, your body feels the repercussions. The body is a mirror of the soul, and when the soul is dimmed, the body dims too.

Energy begins to rise again the moment you take steps toward authenticity. Even the smallest act like writing down an unspoken dream, admitting a hard truth to yourself, or carving out time for what lights you up creates a surge of vitality. This is not coincidence. When you stop resisting your deeper knowing, the nervous system shifts from defense to expansion, and the body reclaims energy once wasted on suppression. Alignment is efficient. Life force is freed instead of being drained.

Purpose is not always a grand mission or world-changing achievement. Sometimes this is simply living in a way that feels congruent with your values. Raising children with presence, tending a garden, speaking honestly, or creating beauty in small ways are all acts of carrying out purpose. These choices may look ordinary from the outside, but they are extraordinary for the inner current of energy they release. The soul does not require fame or recognition, mostly just truth, and once lived, this provides a wellspring of stamina.

When you live aligned with your purpose, fatigue no longer stalks you in the same way. Challenges will come, and effort will still be required, but the strain feels different. Work fueled by meaning invigorates instead of depleting. Even in exhaustion, you feel restored by the clarity of why you are doing what you do. Purpose gives energy context, and in that context, the body and soul cooperate. The river of vitality runs steadily, carrying you through both ease and adversity with a strength that cannot be manufactured by supplements or stimulants.

Fatigue of Inauthentic Living

One of the most common, and least addressed, sources of chronic fatigue is *misalignment*. Living a life that doesn't match who you really are is exhausting. You may look functional on the outside, but deep within, your energy is leaking into the gap between your truth and your reality.

This kind of fatigue doesn't always show up in lab results. It shows up as "Why do I feel so tired when nothing's wrong?" It shows up as procrastination, disengagement, anxiety, and the slow, silent withdrawal from your own life.

The fatigue of inauthentic living is the body's way of demanding honesty. It is not weakness but a signal, a biological protest against the betrayal of your own essence. Every time you say *"yes"* when you mean *"no,"* and each time you swallow your truth to keep the peace, or stay in environments that shrink you, your nervous system spends energy masking instead of flowing. Over weeks and years, that masking becomes as exhausting as running a marathon with no finish line. The cure is not more caffeine or tighter discipline, but courageous alignment and closing the gap between the life you are living and the one your soul keeps asking for.

The Energy of Alignment

The opposite is also true. When you align with purpose, even if difficult and uncertain, energy returns. You rise earlier, breathe deeper, and recover faster. You speak with clarity. You create with conviction. You stop needing as much stimulation because you are powered by *meaning*.

This is the fuel that cannot be faked and does not come from caffeine or hacks. This motivation comes from *knowing who you are and why you are here and choosing to live in that truth*. Even imperfectly.

Alignment creates a feedback loop of vitality. Each step you take in the direction of your soul's truth affirms safety to your nervous system and coherence to your cells. The body interprets authenticity as efficiency. No energy is wasted on pretending, performing, or resisting. Instead, every breath, word, and action begins to reinforce the current of life moving through you. Even when the path is uncertain, the clarity of living congruently becomes a renewable energy source, one that sustains far longer than any external stimulant ever could.

Your Body Responds to Meaning

When you speak from your center, your breath deepens. When you take aligned risks, your immune system strengthens. When you create, serve, build, or express from your soul, not your conditioning, your nervous system stabilizes.

This is not spiritual fluff. This is biology. Meaning *modulates hormones*. Fulfillment lowers cortisol. Purpose sharpens focus. When your life becomes resonant, your energy becomes sustainable.

Signs Your Purpose is Dormant:

• You feel tired even after rest.
• You dread your daily routine.
• You feel like a *"version"* of yourself, not your whole self.
• You rely on external motivation to function.
• You have a deep ache for something more but suppress.

If this is you, your fatigue may not be asking for more supplements, but for a more truthful life. Your purpose does not need to be grandiose, just to be *real*. This lives where your passion meets your compassion. Where your natural gifts meet the world's unmet needs. This can be displayed as parenting with love. Building something beautiful. Teaching, creating, healing, growing, guiding, or protecting. The place where your heart feels most alive. When you reconnect with purpose, you reconnect with yourself. The body, so faithful, so patient, responds with lightness.

Purpose is less about achievement and more about alignment. The sincerity of the song restores energy greater than the size of the stage. Even small daily choices made from truth such as writing a page, planting a seed, cooking with care, or speaking honestly signal to the body that life is worth showing up for. In those moments, fatigue lifts because you are no longer dragging yourself against the current. Instead, you are carried. Meaning is momentum, and once you step in, your biology rises to match your spirit.

How to Reclaim Purpose as Fuel

1. Follow Your Aliveness

• What energizes you, even if this makes no sense?
• What do you lose track of time doing?
• What did you love before the world told you who to be?

2. Audit for Alignment

• Where in your life are you performing or pretending?
• What would you stop doing if you trusted your inner voice?

3. Create Something That Matters to You

• Write. Speak. Cook. Build. Mentor. Paint. Grow.
• Creation is the natural expression of vitality.

4. Serve Something Bigger Than Yourself

• Purpose expands when we give away our excess.
• Ask: Who can I help from my overflow?

5. Let Go of "Shoulds"

• Do not chase what others admire. Chase what *you* feel called to do.
• The nervous system recognizes truth faster than the mind can explain.

Energy is not just in what you consume or expel. This lives in what you *stand for*. When your life begins to reflect your inner knowing, your fatigue becomes fuel. This becomes a signal that something real is waking up inside you. Something worth living for. Something *you came here to do*.

Purpose Reconnection Journal Page

Unearth What Moves You. Align With What is True.

Use these prompts to help rediscover your inner compass. The part of you that knows why you are here and what gives life meaning. Write freely. Do not edit. Let truth rise.

1. What am I naturally drawn to, even if this does not *"make sense"* to others?

_____

_____

2. What energizes me? What drains me?

_____

_____

3. What did I love doing as a child, before anyone told me who to be?

_____

_____

4. What problem do I feel uniquely called to solve, or contribute to solving?

_____

_____

5. What are three moments in life when I felt most alive, clear, and powerful?

_____

_____

6. If I had unlimited energy and no fear, how would I spend my time?

_____

_____

7. What is one small act I can do this week to live more in alignment with that vision?

_____

_____

Your purpose is not something you figure out. This is something you remember.

Soul-Driven Energy Map

Let Purpose Direct Your Vitality

This map helps you visually track what brings energy *into* your life and what depletes energy. Use this to make courageous, soul-aligned adjustments to your schedule, relationships, and creative expression.

Energy Generators (These give me life):

Write down anything that gives you energy, even if subtle or quiet.

− _____
− _____
− _____
− _____

Energy Drains (These consistently wear me down):

Be honest. What do you keep doing that costs too much of your life force?

− _____
− _____
− _____
− _____

Creative Expressions I have Neglected but Miss:

What lights you up that you have not made time for?

− _____
− _____

People Who Amplify My Energy:

Think of those who reflect the real you and leave you feeling better.

− _____
− _____

People or Situations That Diminish My Energy:

Who or what needs boundaries, renegotiation, or release?

− _____
− _____

My Purpose, In One Sentence (for now):

"I feel most alive when I _____
and I believe I am here to _____."

Chapter 13: The Return of Energy

Releasing the Blocks That Keep Vitality Frozen

Energy Gets Trapped

For most people, fatigue is not simply a matter of *"running out"* of energy. This is a matter of energy getting locked away in tension, suppression, and unprocessed experiences. A reason why some days you can sleep eight hours, eat well, and still feel drained is because your nervous system is spending enormous amounts of power keeping things inside you from moving.

When we experience emotional pain, stress, or trauma, the body often responds by tightening, bracing, and creating holding patterns. Over time, these become the default setting. The result? Energy that could go toward creativity, connection, and strength is instead consumed by the quiet, constant labor of holding everything in.

The good news is that what is trapped can be released. Just as ice eventually melts back into water, frozen vitality thaws when we create the right conditions of safety, honesty, and expression. The body holds when we do not feel we have permission to let go. When that permission is granted, often through breath, movement, truth-telling, or the simple act of presence, the nervous system begins to unlock, and energy once bound in tension returns to circulation.

You may notice this release in small ways at first: a spontaneous sigh after speaking from your center, tears flowing unexpectedly in a safe conversation, or laughter erupting after years of seriousness. These are not breakdowns but breakthroughs. They are the body's way of reminding you that energy is meant to move. The more you allow micro-releases, the more often your system remembers how to reset without being forced.

Releasing trapped energy is not about catharsis, but about restoring balance. When vitality flows freely again, healing accelerates. Digestion improves, sleep deepens, immunity strengthens, and creativity awakens. What once felt like chronic exhaustion begins to feel like clarity returning. This is the return of energy. Not manufactured, or borrowed, but remembered from within.

The Emotional Freeze Response

Science calls this *"incomplete stress cycles."* Your body mobilizes energy to respond to a threat, but if that threat cannot be resolved and you are unable to fight, flee, or process, the cycle remains unfinished. That unresolved activation lives on in your muscles, breath, and fascia, keeping you in a subtle but continuous drain.

Signs of a frozen energy state:

• Feeling tired despite rest.

• Tension in jaw, neck, or gut without clear cause.

• Difficulty fully exhaling.

• Brain fog or a sense of "being far away" from your body.

• Emotional numbness.

Unfreezing: The Gentle Thaw

As the emotional body begins to unfreeze, something shifts. Energy comes back in a steady, grounded way. You are no longer wasting the energy you already have or chasing adrenaline highs. You stop spending fuel on internal suppression, and that fuel becomes available for living.

You do not need to be emotionally perfect to reclaim energy. You simply need to be emotionally honest. The soul tires more from being unheard than from doing too much. Even small acts of truth, such as admitting when you feel hurt, expressing gratitude, or saying "no" begin to release the tension dam.

When you allow yourself to feel and move through stored emotion, the nervous system shifts from sympathetic dominance (fight/flight) into parasympathetic repair mode.

This shift:

• Improves mitochondrial function and oxygen use.

• Reduces chronic cortisol output.

• Enhances sleep quality and hormonal balance.

• Frees up glucose and fatty acids for physical energy rather than stress chemistry.

Practices to Invite Energy Back

1. Somatic Breath Release

• Sit or lie down in a safe space.

• Inhale deeply through the nose, exhale with sound through the mouth.

• Visualize tension leaving with the exhale.

• Continue for three to five minutes.

2. Micro-Movements

• Gently shake the hands, roll the shoulders, or sway the hips for one to two minutes.

• These movements signal safety to the body and invite stored activation to move.

3. Expressive Writing

• Set a timer for five to ten minutes.

• Write freely without censoring, allowing thoughts and emotions to spill onto the page.

• When finished, shred or burn the paper. The act of disposal signals completion.

4. Vocal Expression

• Hum, sing, or use vowel sounds to vibrate the throat and chest.

• This stimulates the vagus nerve and can release chest and diaphragm tension.

5. Grounding Through Touch

• Place your palms over your chest or belly and take slow breaths.

• With each inhale, imagine drawing fresh energy up from the earth; with each exhale, release heaviness down into the ground.

• You can also lie on the floor or step outside barefoot, letting your body rest against the support of earth, grass, or stone.

• This restores a sense of safety and connection, allowing frozen energy to discharge gently.

Case Story: The Teacher Who Found Her Voice

Maria, a 42-year-old teacher, came to me complaining of exhaustion despite a clean diet and regular exercise. Within minutes of our first session, I noticed her posture. Her shoulders were slightly hunched, breath shallow, and voice quiet. We worked with simple daily practice: five minutes of humming while rocking side-to-side, followed by ten minutes of unfiltered journaling.

Within three weeks, Maria reported feeling *"more awake"* before noon than she had in years. She began laughing more with her students, sleeping deeper, and even returning to hobbies she had abandoned. Her energy had not come from a supplement or a new workout but had been hiding under years of swallowed words and unspoken boundaries.

Common Blocks to Energy Return

• **Fear of feeling:** Belief that emotions will overwhelm you if felt.

• **Identity attachment:** "I am just a tired person" becomes a self-fulfilling cycle.

• **Lack of safe space:** Without environments where you can express yourself freely, your system stays guarded.

Your Invitation

The return of energy is a relationship, not a single event. You tend to this daily, not by forcing more activity into your life, but by clearing up what no longer needs to be carried. Over time, you will notice that energy becomes something you can trust.

This is the kind of vitality that does not vanish when stress appears but bends without breaking, adapts without abandoning you, and flows without needing to be chased. The energy of alignment, where thoughts, feelings, and actions move together in the same direction.

When you reclaim this energy, fatigue stops being your identity and acts only as a signal. You will have the tools to respond before depletion takes hold.

Chapter 14: The Energy–Environment Connection

Designing Spaces That Feed Your Vitality

Your Environment Is a Constant Conversation

Every second of every day, your body is in dialogue with your surroundings. There is something inside you that listens to the light that hits your eyes, the air that passes through your lungs, the sounds that fill your ears, and the electromagnetic fields that bathe your cells. These inputs determine whether your system feels safe enough to rest and repair or whether to brace, guard, and conserve.

Most fatigue protocols focus on food, movement, and mindset. Your environment, however, can override even the cleanest diet or the most disciplined sleep schedule. You can drink green juice and do breathwork daily, but if you spend your nights under harsh blue light, breathing stale air, or sleeping next to a live router, you are asking your body to heal while still under siege.

The good news? Environmental changes often deliver the fastest, most noticeable returns on energy. When the *"background noise"* drops, your nervous system can finally exhale. Think of your environment as the soil in which your body is planted. Even the most resilient seed will struggle to thrive if the soil is depleted, polluted, or starved of sunlight.

In the same way, your mitochondria, hormones, and nervous system cannot flourish if the space you live and work in is draining rather than nourishing. The body does not separate from environment. We adapt, for better or worse.

This is why purification must extend beyond what you eat and how you move, into how you design the spaces you inhabit. A cluttered, chaotic room translates into subtle stress signals; a quiet, well-ventilated space translates into safety and calm. The presence of natural light, plants, clean water, and fresh air are not luxuries but prerequisites for vitality. When your environment supports you, energy conservation becomes effortless, and fatigue begins to dissolve simply because your body no longer fights your surroundings.

The Biology of Environmental Energy

1. Mitochondria and Light

Your mitochondria are not just fuel processors; they are also light-sensitive engines. Morning sunlight boosts ATP production and sets your circadian clock, while artificial light at night confuses your hormonal cycles and suppresses melatonin.

2. Air Quality and Cellular Load

Indoor air can be two to five times more polluted than outdoor air, often full of dust, mold spores, and off-gassing chemicals. Every breath your body filters is an energy expense, leaving less for movement, thought, and repair.

3. EMFs and Nervous System Tone

Research suggests that high exposure to electromagnetic fields can disrupt voltage-gated calcium channels in cell membranes, contributing to oxidative stress and fatigue. Reducing EMF load can help the body stay in parasympathetic repair mode more often.

4. Clutter and Cognitive Load

Visual clutter increases decision fatigue and cortisol release. When every glance is met with *"unfinished business,"* the nervous system stays on alert.

5. Sound and Nervous System Harmony

Noise pollution taxes the nervous system. Constant background noise, traffic, or electronic hum keeps your body in a low-grade stress response, even if you think you have tuned out. In contrast, natural sounds like birdsong, water, or wind entrain the brain toward calmer frequencies, lowering cortisol and supporting recovery.

6. Temperature and Metabolic Balance

Your body expends enormous energy maintaining internal temperature. Overheated rooms or chronic exposure to air-conditioning can force constant thermoregulation, leaving less energy for healing and performance. Strategically engaging with temperature by welcoming fresh cool air, safe sun exposure, or brief cold exposure can reduce metabolic strain and even build resilience in your mitochondria.

Room-by-Room Energy Audit

Bedroom: Your Charging Station

• Blackout curtains or sleep with an organic mask to block all light.

• Remove Wi-Fi routers, cordless phones, and unnecessary electronics.

• Keep the temperature between 60–67°F for optimal sleep quality.

• Choose natural bedding materials like organic cotton or linen.

Kitchen: Your Fuel Lab

• Install a water filter to remove chlorine, fluoride, heavy metals, and microplastics.

• Replace Teflon or aluminum cookware with stainless steel, glass, or cast iron.

• Keep counters clear: visual order supports digestive calm.

Workspace: Your Command Center

• Position screens at eye level to prevent neck strain.

• Use natural light whenever possible; if not, use full-spectrum bulbs.

• Take a *"visual rest"* every twenty minutes and look twenty feet away for twenty seconds.

• Keep cords, chargers, and routers off the desk surface.

Living Areas: Your Recovery Zones

• Introduce plants like peace lilies or pothos to help filter air.

• Remove or relocate items associated with stress or conflict.

• Use warm light and calming scents in the evening to signal wind-down.

Outdoor Space: Your Natural Battery

• Even a balcony or small yard can become a grounding zone.

• Add a chair for morning sun exposure or barefoot time on grass.

• Keep the space clear of clutter to invite use.

7-Day Environmental Detox Protocol

Day 1: Light Reset

Morning sunlight within thirty minutes of waking; no overhead artificial light after sunset.

Day 2: Air Upgrade

Open windows for ten minutes twice a day; add a HEPA air purifier in your bedroom.

Day 3: EMF Reduction

Unplug or switch off Wi-Fi at night; move your phone out of the bedroom.

Day 4: Clutter Clear

Choose one high-traffic area to declutter completely.

Day 5: Scent and Sound

Introduce calming natural scents (lavender, cedar) and reduce constant background noise.

Day 6: Water Purity

Install a water filter or use a quality countertop filter for drinking and cooking.

Day 7: Emotional Reset

Rearrange one room that holds heavy memories; add an item that inspires peace.

Case Studies

Case 1: EMF-Free Sleep

A client removed their bedroom TV, unplugged the router at night, and switched to an analog alarm clock. Within two weeks, they reported sleeping an hour longer and waking more alert.

Case 2: Mold Awareness

Another client discovered hidden mold behind a piece of furniture. After remediation and adding an air purifier, their daily headaches disappeared, and their afternoon energy slumps eased.

Case 3: The Minimalist Desk

A writer removed piles of books and scattered notes from their workspace, keeping only their laptop and one notebook. They reported a forty percent increase in daily writing output and less mental fatigue.

Case 4: Morning Sun Reset

A young professional committed to stepping outside each morning for ten minutes of sunlight before checking their phone. Within a week, they noticed earlier sleep onset, fewer mid-afternoon crashes, and a more consistent mood throughout the day.

Case 5: Sound Shift

A family living near a busy road began using white noise at night and playing gentle instrumental music in the evenings instead of leaving the TV on for background sound. Their children fell asleep faster, and the parents reported lower evening tension and less irritability.

Case 6: Water Upgrade

A couple replaced their tap water with filtered water for both cooking and drinking. After two weeks, they noticed improved digestion, clearer skin, and reduced bloating. Changes they had not achieved with dietary shifts alone.

Case 7: Scent Reset

A client swapped synthetic air fresheners for natural essential oils like cedarwood and lavender. They reported fewer sinus issues, more restful sleep, and a greater sense of calm when entering their home after work.

Conclusion: You Were Born for Vitality

Remove the Burden. Feed the Fire. Rise Fully Alive.

Fatigue is not your destiny. This was only a messenger. A signal. A compassionate invitation from your body to pause, to listen, and to remember what you are made of.

You were not designed to crawl through life running on fumes. You were built to *radiate*. To move with clarity. To sleep deeply, rise easily, think clearly, and live with a pulse that matches the intelligence of the cosmos flowing through you.

What you have discovered in these pages is more of a reclamation than a protocol. A return to rhythm, to truth, and to living in harmony with the original blueprint encoded within your cells. That blueprint is one of resilience, creativity, and *radiance*.

Remove the Burden, Feed the Fire

Fatigue was always about needing *less of what burdens you*. Less toxicity. Less artificial stimulation. Less pretending. Less inflammation, whether physical, emotional, or spiritual.

We replace fatigue with breath, fruit, laughter, movement, nourishment, purpose, stillness, and truth. The elemental forces that rebuild you from the inside out.

You do not need synthetic energy. You need *permission to be natural again*. To live in a way that honors the sacredness of your biology and the wisdom of your soul.

When you remember this, fatigue transforms from an enemy into a guide. Every dip in energy becomes feedback, every symptom an invitation to realign, and every moment of renewal a reminder that your body is not against you but always working for you. Vitality is not something you chase but is what rises naturally when you remove what dulls you and allow life's current to move freely through you. To live this way is not only to heal yourself but to become a living signal of possibility for others, showing that radiant energy is our birthright, waiting to be reclaimed.

What Fatigue Immunity Feels Like

Fatigue immunity involves being *in rhythm*. When your body is no longer burdened, when your purpose is no longer suppressed, and when your life reflects who you really are, energy flows. You do not force; you simply clear the way.

Fatigue immunity means you no longer live tired. You will still have days of effort, seasons of intensity, and moments when rest is required. Instead of exhaustion being your baseline, though, fatigue becomes a signal: *a whisper that you need recalibration, not a sentence you must endure.* In this state, recovery is swift, and energy flows from alignment, not adrenaline.

This kind of vitality bends with stress without breaking, adapts to challenge without collapse, and restores with the simple practices you have woven into daily life. You stop fearing that energy will vanish and start trusting the return, because your body and spirit are now in conversation. Fatigue immunity feels like freedom. The freedom to live fully, to create boldly, and to meet life with presence rather than depletion.

The end of fatigue feels like:

• Waking up without dread.

• Breathing without tension.

• Moving without hesitation.

• Creating without burning out.

• Digesting with ease.

• Thinking with clarity.

• Resting deeply without guilt.

• Saying no without apology.

• Saying yes to your life.

• Knowing that energy is no longer a currency you chase but a presence you *embody*.

Closing Integration Practice

Anchor the Journey. Embody the Shift.

Time Required: 15–20 minutes.

Setting: Quiet space, nature if possible, barefoot or grounded.

1. Ground and Breathe

• Stand or sit with your feet planted.
• Inhale deeply through the nose for a count of four.
• Hold for four.
• Exhale slowly for eight.
• Repeat for five to ten rounds, relaxing your shoulders, jaw, and belly.

2. Speak Intentions Out Loud

Affirm the shift you have made. Speak one or more of the following:

• "I am no longer available for depletion."
• "I honor my energy as sacred."
• "I choose rhythm over rush. Alignment over force."
• "My vitality is rising. My light is returning."

3. Feel the Fire

Close your eyes and place a hand over your heart or solar plexus. Visualize a warm, steady glow building inside you. Not a spark that flickers, but a *fire that stays*. Let this radiate outward and allow your body to remember this as *home*.

4. Commit to Your Non-Negotiables

Whisper or write: "What do I now know I must protect?"

• My sleep rhythm.
• My morning light and breathwork.
• My boundaries.
• My fruit-based diet.
• My movement practice.

5. Close with Intention

Say silently or aloud:

"I walk forward with light in my cells and clarity in my steps. I am immune to fatigue because I live in harmony. This is my new way."

Final Reflection Journal Page

Use this page to capture the essence of your journey. Let this be raw, imperfect, and real. You can revisit this as your baseline or reread whenever you feel lost or low.

What have I learned about my body's true nature?

_____

_____

What was one belief about fatigue I have released?

_____

_____

What feels different in me now, physically, emotionally, or spiritually?

_____

_____

What is my body asking for more of moving forward?

_____

_____

What am I no longer willing to tolerate in my life?

_____

_____

What energy practices do I want to protect with devotion?

_____

_____

If I could send one message to my future self, this would be:

_____

_____

This is your life force.
Reclaimed.
Guarded.
Treasured.
From this place, you rise.

Resource Appendix

Support for the Ongoing Journey

This is a curated collection of practices, tools, and modalities you can explore to deepen your fatigue immunity journey.

Core Daily Anchors

• Morning sun exposure and nasal breathwork.
• Daily raw fruit and/or green juice.
• Movement (lymphatic, cardio, grounding).
• Cold therapy, dry brushing, sauna or rebounding.
• Intermittent fasting or fruit-only mornings.
• Digital sunsets (screens off one hour before bed).
• Parasympathetic activation (breath, nature, stillness).

Detoxification Tools

• Colonics or enemas.
• Herbal parasite protocols (e.g., wormwood, clove, black walnut).
• Heavy metal detox support (cilantro, spirulina, fulvic minerals).
• Castor oil packs over liver or abdomen.
• Mold detox (binders, glutathione, air purifiers).

Plant-Based Energy Allies

• Beets, watermelon, citrus, greens, herbs, and sprouts.
• Sea moss, dulse, chlorella, adaptogens (ashwagandha, reishi).
• High-mineral foods (coconut water, celery juice, shilajit).
• Anti-inflammatory staples (ginger, turmeric, flaxseed).

Somatic & Emotional Release Modalities

• Breathwork (Wim Hof, conscious connected, box breathing).
• TRE (Tension & Trauma Release Exercises).
• Ecstatic dance or intuitive movement.
• Journaling, voice note venting, unsent letters.
• Therapy, EMDR, somatic experiencing, inner child work.

Sacred Sleep Supports

• Blue-light blockers and red-light bulbs.
• Magnesium glycinate or topical magnesium spray.
• Herbal sleep teas (skullcap, chamomile, passionflower).
• Nightly wind-down rituals (yoga, stretching, low-stim music).

Thirty-Day Fatigue Immunity Protocol

One Month to Reset Your Rhythm, Restore Your Energy, and Remember Your Fire

This thirty-day protocol combines cleansing, nourishment, movement, and emotional recalibration. Each week builds on the last, layering simplicity and sustainability.

Week 1: Clear the Static

Focus: Open detox pathways, hydrate, simplify.

Daily Essentials:

- Hydrate upon waking (lemon water or cucumber juice).

- Eliminate dairy, caffeine, refined sugar, and fried foods.

- Eat raw fruits before noon (mono meals ideal).

- Add one raw salad per day.

- Move for thirty minutes: walk, bounce, stretch.

- Dry brush or use sauna if available.

- Sleep before 10:00 PM.

Bonus: Begin journaling: "Where am I tired because I am not being true?"

Week 2: Feed the Fire

Focus: Deep cellular nourishment.

Daily Essentials:

- Add 16 oz green juice daily (celery, cucumber, parsley, lemon).

- Incorporate beets or beet juice (for nitric oxide).

- High-raw eating: fruits, veggies, healthy fats, sprouts.

- Eat dinner by 7:00 PM.

- 3x/week breathwork sessions (ten to fifteen minutes).

- Forty-five minutes of daily movement.

- Digital sunset (no screens one hour before bed).

Bonus: Speak one boundary or truth aloud this week.

Week 3: Release & Restore

Focus: Lymphatic flow & emotional clearing.

Daily Essentials:

• Practice rebounding or lymphatic movement fifteen minutes a day.

• Take one full day of juice fasting or fruit mono-meal.

• Integrate one grief or rage release session (cry, scream, write).

• Take magnesium or adaptogenic herbs in the evening.

• Use castor oil pack 2x this week over liver.

• Sleep with zero EMF (Wi-Fi off, phone away).

Bonus: Ask: "What have I been carrying that is not mine?"

Week 4: Align & Energize

Focus: Soul clarity & energy preservation.

Daily Essentials:

• Anchor morning and evening rituals.

• Replace *"to-do"* mindset with *"to-feel"* presence.

• Create something: *write, sing, garden, teach.*

• Serve someone with your overflow.

• Refine movement practice: *powerful yet easeful.*

• Reflect on purpose: *"What is emerging in me?"*

• Choose one lifestyle upgrade to make permanent.

Bonus: Write a letter to your future, fatigue-free self.

Meal Plans & Recipes for Mitochondrial Health

Fuel the Fire. Feed the Cell. Live Alkaline.

Your mitochondria are micropower plants and they respond instantly to what you feed them. These meal plans and recipes are rich in hydration, enzymes, structured glucose, trace minerals, and alkalinity. Each recipe supports energy production, oxygenation, and inflammation reduction.

Instead of seeing food as calories alone, begin to observe information in the food you consume. The coded messages that either signal your cells to burn clean or to clog and corrode. Fresh fruits, leafy greens, sprouted grains, nuts, seeds, and vibrant vegetables carry electrical life force that mitochondria translate into steady, sustainable energy. By contrast, processed foods, chemical additives, and animal-heavy meals generate metabolic waste that forces mitochondria to fight through sludge just to keep your lights on. The difference in how you feel is not subtle; this is the difference between living on fumes and living on fire.

Hydration, color diversity, and ease of digestion are the pillars of these recipes. Meals should leave you feeling lighter, clearer, and more alert, not heavy or sluggish. Think of juices that deliver structured water and minerals directly into your cells; salads that combine bitter greens with citrus to awaken the liver; bowls of quinoa or millet paired with steamed vegetables and herbs that fuel without inflammation. This is not restriction but restoration, a return to the food that reminds your body how to thrive.

Foundational Guidelines for Fatigue-Free Eating

• **Begin your day with fruit or green juice**: always hydrating, never heavy.

• **Avoid mucus-forming foods:** dairy, gluten, eggs, oils, processed animal products.

• **Prioritize raw foods:** for enzymatic repair.

• **No food after 7:00 PM**: let digestion rest and hormones reset.

• **Simplify meals** (2–5 ingredients max): to preserve digestive energy.

• **Chew thoroughly and eat mindfully**: digestion begins in the mouth.

• **Stay mineral-rich:** include sea vegetables, leafy greens, and unrefined salts to replenish electrolytes and support mitochondrial function.

Sample Daily Meal Plan (High Raw / Energy Focused)

Morning (7:00–9:00 AM):

• 16 oz lemon water or cucumber juice.

• Option 1: Fresh papaya with lime.

• Option 2: Fruit mono-meal (e.g., watermelon, mango).

• Optional: Sea moss gel with cinnamon].

Late Morning (10:00–11:30 AM):

• Green Juice (celery, cucumber, cilantro, lime, green apple).

• Optional: Spirulina shot or coconut water.

Lunch (12:30–2:00 PM):

•Big salad with mixed greens, arugula, sprouts, avocado, cucumber, and pumpkin seeds.

• Dressing: lemon, tahini, ginger, red Alaea sea salt, water blend.

• Side: Steamed beets or sweet potato.

Afternoon Snack (3:30–4:30 PM):

• Green smoothie (banana, spinach, coconut water, flaxseed, spirulina).

• Or: Handful of berries with coconut yogurt.

Dinner (5:30–6:30 PM):

• Light amaranth or millet bowl with steamed broccoli, kale, and chickpeas.

• Herbs and anti-fatigue spices: turmeric, cumin, black seed.

• Herbal tea (nettles, ginger, tulsi).

Fatigue-Fighting Recipes

Revive Green Juice
Energizing + Alkalizing

- 1 head celery
- 1 cucumber
- 1 small green apple
- ½ bunch cilantro
- 1 lime, peeled
- → Juice and serve immediately

Mitochondria Smoothie
Oxygen-rich + Antioxidant boost

- 2 cups wild blueberries & cherries
- 1 tsp sea moss gel
- 1 tbsp ground flaxseed
- 1 cup coconut water
- → **Blend until creamy**

Liver-Loving Salad
Bitter, mineral-rich, and blood cleansing

- Arugula
- Dandelion greens
- Cucumber
- Radish
- Sprouts
- Lemon-tahini dressing with a dash of cayenne
- → **Add avocado or hemp seeds for healthy fats**

Anti-Fatigue Broth
Deep mineral and nervous system reset

- 2 celery stalks
- 1 large carrot
- ½ sweet potato
- 1 handful parsley
- 1 strip kombu or dulse
- Ginger and turmeric root slices
- Sea salt, bay leaf
- → **Simmer in filtered water for 45 min. Strain. Sip slowly.**

Supplement & Detox Toolkit

Support for Mitochondrial Health, Detox Pathways, and Energy Resilience

Supplements are not substitutes for rhythm, rest, and real food—but they can powerfully assist your body's return to vitality. Below is a curated toolkit of foundational supplements and detox support formulas to enhance mitochondrial function, reduce inflammation, and remove cellular waste.

Mitochondrial Support

(Use daily or in focused energy-rebuilding phases)

• **CoQ10 (Ubiquinol)** – Supports mitochondrial energy output and cardiovascular health.

• **PQQ** – Encourages mitochondrial biogenesis (creation of new mitochondria).

• **NAD+ Precursors (NMN or NR)** – Boosts cellular repair and mitochondrial performance.

• **Magnesium Glycinate or Malate** – Essential for over 300 enzymatic reactions, including ATP production.

• **Acetyl-L-Carnitine** – Enhances fat metabolism and mental clarity.

Liver & Lymph Detox Support

(Use during and after cleansing protocols or toxic exposures)

• **Milk Thistle (silymarin)** – Regenerates and protects liver cells.

• **Dandelion Root** – Bile flow, liver support, mild diuretic.

• **Burdock Root** – Blood purifier and lymph mover.

• **Red Clover or Cleavers** – Lymphatic drainage and skin support.

• **Castor Oil Packs** – External detox tool to stimulate lymph and liver detox.

Heavy Metal & Mold Detox Support

(Use under guidance during chelation or environmental exposure detox)

• **Chlorella + Cilantro (combo)** – Bind and mobilize heavy metals.

• **Activated Charcoal** – Absorbs mycotoxins and gut endotoxins (short-term use).

• **Zeolite (clinoptilolite)** – Binds to and removes toxic compounds.

• **Bentonite Clay (internal or external)** – Natural binding agent for toxins.

• **Glutathione (liposomal)** – Master antioxidant and cellular protector.

Respiratory + Oxygen Support

(Use for fatigue related to poor oxygenation or chronic congestion)

• **Beetroot Extract or Juice Powder** – Boosts nitric oxide and blood flow.

• **L-Arginine or Citrulline** – Supports nitric oxide and vascular flexibility.

• **N-Acetyl Cysteine (NAC)** – Clears mucus and supports glutathione production.

• **Mullein Leaf** – Herbal lung tonic.

• **Cordyceps Mushroom** – Oxygen efficiency and endurance enhancer.

Core Energy Formulas

(Build your own protocol or work with a practitioner to personalize)

• **B-Complex (methylated)** – Nerve support and energy metabolism.

• **Vitamin C (liposomal or whole food-based)** – Adrenal support and antioxidant.

• **Omega-3s (algae-based)** – Brain and mitochondrial membrane integrity.

• **Electrolyte powder (without artificial sweeteners)** – Hydration and mineral balance.

• **Adaptogens (Ashwagandha, Rhodiola, Holy Basil)** – Nervous system resilience.

Supplements work best when your body is ready to receive them. This means while hydrated, open, and supported by a clean lifestyle. Start slow, listen deeply, and track your shifts.

Fatigue Immunity Journal Pages

Track Your Truth. Witness Your Rise. Stay in Rhythm.

These daily and weekly journaling pages are designed to help you observe patterns, recalibrate your practices, and stay intimately connected with your energy. They offer structure with freedom, so your healing can become a lifestyle, not just a phase.

Daily Energy Clarity Log

Date: _____

Sleep Hours Last Night: _____

Overall Energy Level (1–10): _____

Morning Check-In

How do I feel physically?

How do I feel emotionally?

What is one thing I can do today to support my energy?

Midday Check-In

Did I hydrate today? Y / N

Did I move? Y / N

Have I eaten mostly plant-based, clean foods? Y / N

How is my breath right now, shallow or deep?

Evening Check-In

What was the most energizing moment of my day?

_____

What drained me? Did I allow more or present a challenge?

_____

One thing I am proud of today:

_____

Something I want to do differently tomorrow:

_____

My body is asking for:

☐ Rest
☐ More movement
☐ Emotional release
☐ Nourishment
☐ Silence
☐ Connection

Weekly Reflection Page

Week of: _____

What patterns of energy depletion did I notice this week?

_____

_____

What gave me energy consistently?

_____

What boundaries or shifts did I make, or need to make?

_____

What did my body teach me this week?

_____

What is one non-negotiable I will commit to for the coming week?

_____

A mantra or intention for the next 7 days:

FAQs: Caffeine, Kids, Shift Work & More

Real-Life Questions. Grounded Guidance.

This section offers practical answers to the most common fatigue-related questions, rooted in the principles of this book, yet flexible enough to honor where you are.

Q: Do I have to give up caffeine completely?

A: Not necessarily but understand that caffeine is a *borrowed currency* that does not create energy. This stimulates your stress response and exhausts your adrenals over time. If you are healing from chronic fatigue, consider:

• Switching to green tea or yerba mate (lower caffeine, gentler lift).

• Delaying caffeine until after breakfast and morning hydration.

• Taking a thirty-day caffeine break to reset your natural energy baseline.

• Replacing morning coffee with warm lemon water, green juice, or beet juice.

Remember: the goal is to rebuild trust in your natural energy cycle.

Q: How can I stay energized while raising young children?

A: Fatigue in parenting is real, and not always avoidable. Even amidst chaos, you can anchor into nourishment and rhythm:

• Prioritize hydration: fruit, smoothies, mineral-rich drinks.

• Batch-cook plant-based meals you can grab and go (e.g., black eye pea & sweet potato bowls, smoothies, veggie stews).

• Involve your kids in movement: dance, nature walks, breathwork.

• Sleep when they sleep (at least once a week!).

• Trade childcare or cleaning help where possible. *Community equals capacity.*

You cannot pour from an empty cup. Fill your cup in sips if you must.

Q: What if I work nights or rotating shifts?

A: Shift work challenges circadian health, but with awareness, you can protect your energy:

• Wear blue-light blocking glasses on night shifts.

• Keep your sleeping space completely dark and cool during daylight rest.

• Stick to consistent eating windows, even if your wake time fluctuates.

• Use adaptogens like ashwagandha, holy basil, and reishi to support cortisol regulation.

• Hydrate more aggressively. Shift work depletes minerals fast.

You may be outside the norm, but your body still loves rhythm. Give it one, even if unconventional.

Q: What is the best thing to eat when I feel an energy crash coming?

A: Reach for *hydrating, enzymatic fuel,* not sugar or stimulants.

Top options:

• Green juice or beet juice.

• Coconut water with lime.

• Fruit mono-meal (papaya, berries, grapes).

• Mineral broth with herbs and seaweed.

• Smoothie with wild blueberries, dates, sea moss, and Tonic Alchemy.

Avoid:

• Processed snacks

• Baked goods

• Energy drinks

• Fried or animal-heavy foods

Q: How do I know if I am doing "enough"?

A: The body will tell you. Look for:

Signs of progress:

• You wake with more ease

• Less bloat, brain fog, or food cravings

• More emotional stability

• Deeper sleep, fewer crashes

• Increased clarity or desire to move/create

   If you are not there yet, simplify. Go back to fruit, water, breath, and rest. This combination works.

Q: What if I fall off track?

A: Then you begin again. Fatigue immunity is not about perfection—it's about *pattern change*. Your body is always willing to heal when you return to the rhythm.

• Choose one practice and recommit.

• Clean one meal, breathe for five minutes, drink one juice.

• Let the return be gentle. Let the journey be honest.

Your body is waiting for you. Begin again today.

Final Blessing

For the Body That Chose to Rise Again

May you remember that fatigue was never your identity, only a phase of forgetting. May your breath become your guide, never labored, always wise. May you be reminded that every exhalation is a release of what no longer belongs, and each inhale is the acceptance of life in pure form. You exhale waste. You inhale *vitalization*.

May your lungs stay soft, your legs strong, and your heart open. May your movement be prayer and your rest be praise. When you run, whether across earth or through experience, may your breath never burn from exhaustion, but flow as a rhythm that carries you beyond limits.

You were not built to burn out. You were not meant to crawl through life saving scraps of energy. You are not here to cope. You are here to *glow*.

May your mitochondria sing with clean fuel. May your thoughts be aligned with truth. May your food be alive and your sleep be sacred. May your boundaries protect your peace. May your emotions move like rivers, never dammed, and never drowned. May your spirit, after all you have unlearned, rest in rhythm once more.

You are not fragile. You are luminous. The moment you chose to trust your body again, you began the return.

This is not the end of a book. This is the beginning of a new way to live. A life where fatigue fades, and vitality becomes the breath that carries you home.

About the Author

Jesse Jacoby is a dedicated father, expressionist, and advocate for compassion, equanimity, and purity. He expends energy adventuring in forests, creating, learning, playing, and writing.

Jesse is the founder and CEO of Soulspire: The Healing Playground (*soulspire.com*). This is a biohacking and purification center with locations near Lake Tahoe in Truckee, CA, and in Nevada City, CA.

He is also the founder of the Global School of Purification (*schoolofpurity.com*), which is an educational course instructing how to regenerate health in the body and providing certifications for global purification specialists.

In addition, Jesse is the co-founder of Substance Shield (*substanceshield.com*), an all organic, food-derived, wild-crafted and botanical supplementation product line designed to help users replenish their body after experimenting with drugs and other substances.

Jesse is the author of The Raw Cure: Healing Beyond Medicine (1st & 2nd Editions), The Way Knows: Trusting Divine Orchestration, Where Galaxies Kiss the Earth, The High Life, Windsdom: Wisdom from the Wind, Sovereign Biology, Immune to Fatigue, The Purification Principle, Modern Human Conditions, You Are Not Powerless, Forged: The Twelve Foundations of Manhood, Gaia Speaks, Eating Plant-Based: The New Health Paradigm, & My Quest to Conquer What Matters.

He also co-founded Little Manifestors Publishing and has authored over thirty children's books.

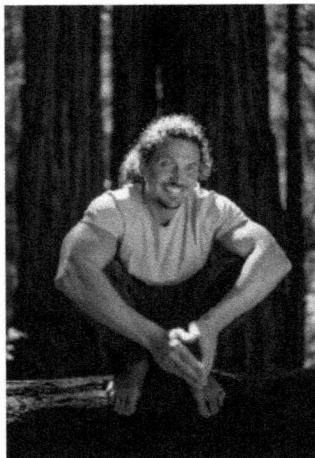

Jesse@soulspire.com

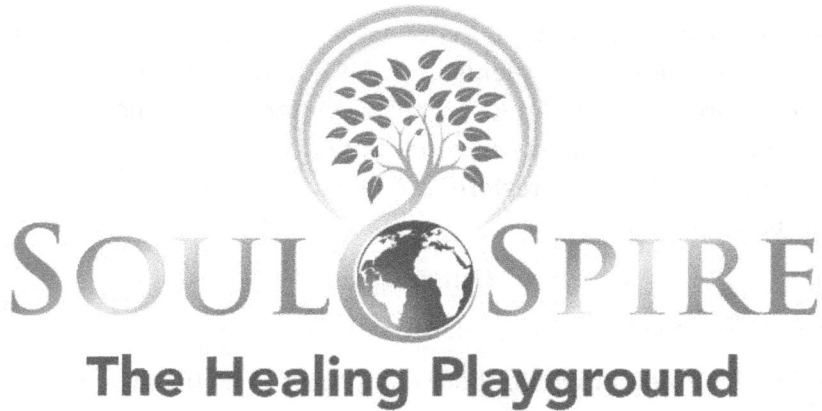

SOUL⊕SPIRE

The Healing Playground

Soulspire is a biohacking and purification offering with centers located in Truckee, CA, and Nevada City, CA which provides each of the biohacking tools suggested in this guide for regenerating the body before and after substance use.

Access the site www.soulspire.com

Substance Shield
Ally of the Aftermath

Substance Shield is a botanical supplement line born from the wisdom of The High Life, a guide for conscious living in a chemically saturated world. Our products exist to support the body's resilience before and after exposure to substances, offering tools of renewal, not judgment. Whether facing pharmaceutical fallout, recreational recovery, or environmental residue, our mission is to replenish what modern life strips away.

Every formula is organic, vegan, wild-harvested, and crafted from whole foods, roots, and ancient botanicals designed to support detoxification pathways, restore depleted micronutrients, and aid in cellular resilience.

Our Mission

- To honor the human experience without shame.

- To offer nourishment to those navigating a chemically compromised world.

- To replenish what substances diminish, without ever promoting their use.

- To be the shield when the soul forgets we have one.

We believe everyone deserves to recover their clarity, reclaim their vitality, and rise stronger after the storm. Whether you have danced with the edge or been caught in the crossfire, Substance Shield is your ally of the aftermath.

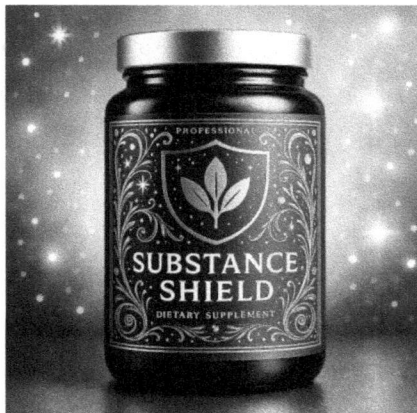

www.substanceshield.com

Bibliography

Intro:
- Brazier, Brendan. *Thrive: The Vegan Nutrition Guide to Optimal Performance in Sports and Life*. Da Capo Press, 2008.
- Hanh, Thich Nhat. *Peace Is Every Step: The Path of Mindfulness in Everyday Life*. Bantam, 1991.
- Hotema, Hilton. *Man's Higher Consciousness*. Health Research Books, 1962.
- Roll, Rich. *Finding Ultra: Rejecting Middle Age, Becoming One of the World's Fittest Men, and Discovering Myself*. Harmony Books, 2012.
- Rudd, Richard. *The Gene Keys: Embracing Your Higher Purpose*. Eden Press, 2013.

Chapter 1:
- Campbell, Bruce, and Michael F. Holick. *Mitochondria and the Future of Medicine: The Key to Understanding Disease, Chronic Illness, Aging, and Life Itself*. Chelsea Green Publishing, 2018.
- Chan, Wing-Tsit, translator. *The Tao Te Ching*. By Laozi, Princeton University Press, 1963. Cutler, David Neal. *The Role of Environmental Toxins in Mitochondrial Dysfunction and Disease*. Elsevier, 2017.
- Naviaux, Robert K. "Metabolic Features of the Cell Danger Response." *Mitochondrion*, vol. 16, 2014, pp. 7–17.
- Sapolsky, Robert M. *Why Zebras Don't Get Ulcers: The Acclaimed Guide to Stress, Stress-Related Diseases, and Coping*. Holt Paperbacks, 2004.
- Wallace, Douglas C. "Mitochondria and Cancer." *Nature Reviews Cancer*, vol. 12, no. 10, 2012, pp. 685–98.
- Zimmerman, Joseph. *Qi Gong and the Healing Arts: Ancient Practices for Modern Health*. Inner Traditions, 2015.

Chapter 2:
- Caldecott, Todd. *Ayurveda: The Divine Science of Life*. Elsevier, 2006.
- Frawley, David. *Ayurveda and the Mind: The Healing of Consciousness*. Lotus Press, 1997.
- Kaptchuk, Ted J. *The Web That Has No Weaver: Understanding Chinese Medicine*. McGraw-Hill, 2000.
- Maté, Gabor. *When the Body Says No: Exploring the Stress-Disease Connection*. Vintage Canada, 2003.
- Sapolsky, Robert M. *Why Zebras Don't Get Ulcers: The Acclaimed Guide to Stress, Stress-Related Diseases, and Coping*. Holt Paperbacks, 2004.
- Satchinanda, Swami. *The Yoga Sutras of Patanjali*. Integral Yoga Publications, 1978.
- Walker, Matthew. *Why We Sleep: Unlocking the Power of Sleep and Dreams*. Scribner, 2017.
- Wallace, B. Alan. *The Attention Revolution: Unlocking the Power of the Focused Mind*. Wisdom Publications, 2006.

Chapter 3:
- Campbell, Andrew W. "Mold, Mycotoxins, and Chronic Illness: The Hidden Connection." *Alternative Therapies in Health and Medicine*, vol. 20, no. 6, 2014, pp. 48–52.
- Cutler, David Neal. *The Role of Environmental Toxins in Mitochondrial Dysfunction and Disease*. Elsevier, 2017.

- Dietrich, Daniel R., et al. *Human Exposure to Environmental Chemicals and Their Impact on Health*. Springer, 2019.
- Havas, Magda. "Electromagnetic Hypersensitivity: Biological Effects of Low-Level Exposure to EMFs." *Environmental Reviews*, vol. 7, no. 2, 2000, pp. 173–204.
- Klinghardt, Dietrich. "Chronic Infections as Hidden Cause of Chronic Fatigue and Illness." *Journal of Nutritional and Environmental Medicine*, vol. 11, no. 3, 2001, pp. 241–50.
- Martinez, Jose L. *Antibiotics and Antibiotic Resistance Genes in Natural Environments*. Springer, 2009.
- Pizzorno, Joseph. *The Toxin Solution: How Hidden Poisons in the Air, Water, Food, and Products We Use Are Destroying Our Health—And What We Can Do to Fix It*. HarperOne, 2017.
- Shoemaker, Ritchie C. *Surviving Mold: Life in the Era of Dangerous Buildings*. Otter Bay Books, 2010.
- Seneff, Stephanie. "Glyphosate, Pathways to Modern Diseases II: Celiac Sprue and Gluten Intolerance." *Interdisciplinary Toxicology*, vol. 6, no. 4, 2013, pp. 159–84.
- Yehuda, Rachel, and Linda M. Bierer. "The Relevance of Epigenetics to PTSD: Implications for the Long-Term Effects of Trauma." *Biological Psychiatry*, vol. 70, no. 4, 2011, pp. 308–14.

Chapter 4:
- Ballentine, Rudolph. *Radical Healing: Integrating the World's Great Therapeutic Traditions to Create a New Transformative Medicine*. Harmony Books, 2000.
- Bratman, Steven, and David Knight. *Encyclopedia of Natural Medicine*. Prima Publishing, 1999.
- Buhner, Stephen Harrod. *Herbal Antibiotics: Natural Alternatives for Treating Drug-Resistant Bacteria*. Storey Publishing, 2012.
- Chia, Mantak. *Chi Nei Tsang: Internal Organs Chi Massage*. Destiny Books, 2007.
- Chevallier, Andrew. *Encyclopedia of Herbal Medicine*. DK Publishing, 2016.
- Gittleman, Ann Louise. *Living Beauty Detox Program: The Revolutionary Diet for Each and Every Season of a Woman's Life*. HarperOne, 2000.
- Holford, Patrick. *The Detox Cookbook: The Complete Guide to Detoxing Safely & Effectively*. Piatkus, 1998.
- Hyman, Mark. *The UltraMind Solution: Fix Your Broken Brain by Healing Your Body First*. Scribner, 2008.
- Kuhn, Merrily. *Kuhn's Herbal Therapy and Supplements: A Scientific and Traditional Approach*. Lippincott Williams & Wilkins, 2000.
- Pitchford, Paul. *Healing with Whole Foods: Asian Traditions and Modern Nutrition*. North Atlantic Books, 2002.
- Shoemaker, Ritchie C. *Surviving Mold: Life in the Era of Dangerous Buildings*. Otter Bay Books, 2010.
- Walker, Matthew. *Why We Sleep: Unlocking the Power of Sleep and Dreams*. Scribner, 2017.

Chapter 5:
- Brazier, Brendan. *Thrive: The Vegan Nutrition Guide to Optimal Performance in Sports and Life*. Da Capo Press, 2008.
- Campbell, T. Colin, and Thomas M. Campbell II. *The China Study: The Most Comprehensive Study of Nutrition Ever Conducted and the Startling Implications for Diet, Weight Loss, and Long-Term Health*. BenBella Books, 2006.

- Esselstyn, Caldwell B. *Prevent and Reverse Heart Disease: The Revolutionary, Scientifically Proven, Nutrition-Based Cure*. Avery, 2007.
- Jones, Andrew M. "Dietary Nitrate Supplementation and Exercise Performance." *Sports Medicine*, vol. 44, suppl. 1, 2014, pp. 35–45.
- Miller, G. D., et al. "Dietary Patterns, Antioxidants and Mitochondrial Function." *Nutrition Reviews*, vol. 71, no. 1, 2013, pp. 34–45.
- Polizzi, Katherine M., and Nathan S. Bryan. "Nitric Oxide and Clinical Nutrition: Focus on the Cardiovascular System." *Nutrition Research*, vol. 33, no. 12, 2013, pp. 872–84.
- Roll, Rich. *Finding Ultra: Rejecting Middle Age, Becoming One of the World's Fittest Men, and Discovering Myself*. Harmony Books, 2012.
- Williams, Melvin H. *Nutrition for Health, Fitness, and Sport*. McGraw-Hill, 2012.

Chapter 6:
- Barnes, Michael, et al. "Intermittent Fasting and Human Metabolic Health." *Journal of Clinical Investigation*, vol. 130, no. 2, 2020, pp. 573–81.
- Longo, Valter, and Satchidananda Panda. "Fasting, Circadian Rhythms, and Time-Restricted Feeding in Healthy Lifespan." *Cell Metabolism*, vol. 23, no. 6, 2016, pp. 1048–59.
- Mattson, Mark P., and Rafael de Cabo. "Effects of Intermittent Fasting on Health, Aging, and Disease." *New England Journal of Medicine*, vol. 381, no. 26, 2019, pp. 2541–51.
- Müller, Matthias J., et al. "Short-Term Fasting and Energy Metabolism: A Systematic Review." *Nutrition, Metabolism & Cardiovascular Diseases*, vol. 27, no. 12, 2017, pp. 1033–47.
- Ohsumi, Yoshinori. "Historical Landmarks of Autophagy Research." *Cell Research*, vol. 24, 2014, pp. 9–23.
- Sahlin, Kent, et al. "Juice Fasting and Detoxification: Effects on Inflammation and Oxidative Stress." *Complementary Therapies in Medicine*, vol. 25, 2016, pp. 93–99.
- Sears, Barry. *The Zone: A Dietary Road Map*. HarperCollins, 1995.
- Tinsley, Grant M., and Paul M. La Bounty. "Effects of Intermittent Fasting on Body Composition and Clinical Health Markers in Humans." *Nutrition Reviews*, vol. 73, no. 10, 2015, pp. 661–74.
- Wilcox, Ralph. *Fasting and Feasting in the Bible and the Qur'an: A Comparative Study*. Routledge, 2014.

Chapter 7:
- Booth, Frank W., et al. "Lack of Exercise Is a Major Cause of Chronic Diseases." *Comprehensive Physiology*, vol. 2, no. 2, 2012, pp. 1143–1211.
- Calabrese, Edward J., and Linda A. Baldwin. "Hormesis: The Dose-Response Revolution." *Annual Review of Pharmacology and Toxicology*, vol. 43, 2003, pp. 175–97.
- Hoffman-Goetz, Laurie, and Candace M. Pedersen. "Exercise and the Lymphatic System: Implications for Disease Prevention and Treatment." *Canadian Journal of Physiology and Pharmacology*, vol. 77, no. 8, 1999, pp. 555–64.
- Holloszy, John O. "Regulation of Mitochondrial Biogenesis in Cells and Tissues." *Biochimica et Biophysica Acta (BBA) – Molecular Cell Research*, vol. 1410, no. 2, 1999, pp. 1–16.
- Mattson, Mark P. "Energy Intake, Exercise, and Brain Health." *Ageing Research Reviews*, vol. 11, no. 3, 2012, pp. 307–20.
- McCall, Tim. *Yoga as Medicine: The Yogic Prescription for Health and Healing*. Bantam, 2007.
Sapolsky, Robert M. *Why Zebras Don't Get Ulcers: The Acclaimed Guide to Stress, Stress-Related Diseases, and Coping*. Holt Paperbacks, 2004.

• Westcott, Wayne L. *Building Strength and Stamina*. Human Kinetics, 2015.

Chapter 8:
• Bjorvatn, Bjørn, et al. "The Role of Light in the Human Circadian System." *Sleep Medicine Reviews*, vol. 7, no. 1, 2003, pp. 59–72.
• Bryant, Penelope A., et al. "Circadian Rhythms and the Immune System." *Immunology and Cell Biology*, vol. 82, no. 6, 2004, pp. 479–86.
• Iliff, Jeffrey J., et al. "A Paravascular Pathway Facilitates CSF Flow Through the Brain Parenchyma and the Clearance of Interstitial Solutes, Including Amyloid β." *Science Translational Medicine*, vol. 4, no. 147, 2012, pp. 147ra111.
• Irwin, Michael R. "Sleep and Inflammation: Partners in Sickness and in Health." *Nature Reviews Immunology*, vol. 19, 2019, pp. 702–15.
• Panda, Satchidananda. *The Circadian Code: Lose Weight, Supercharge Your Energy, and Transform Your Health from Morning to Midnight*. Rodale Books, 2018.
• Rea, Mark S. *Light, Sleep, and Circadian Rhythms: An Integrative Approach*. Springer, 2010.
• Samuels, Charles. "Sleep, Recovery, and Performance: The New Frontier in High-Performance Athletics." *Neurologic Clinics*, vol. 26, no. 1, 2008, pp. 169–80.
• Walker, Matthew. *Why We Sleep: Unlocking the Power of Sleep and Dreams*. Scribner, 2017.

Chapter 9:
• Campbell, T. Colin, and Thomas M. Campbell II. *The China Study: The Most Comprehensive Study of Nutrition Ever Conducted and the Startling Implications for Diet, Weight Loss, and Long-Term Health*. BenBella Books, 2006.
• Hyman, Mark. *The UltraMind Solution: Fix Your Broken Brain by Healing Your Body First*. Scribner, 2008.
• Lipton, Bruce H. *The Biology of Belief: Unleashing the Power of Consciousness, Matter & Miracles*. Hay House, 2015.
• Maté, Gabor. *When the Body Says No: Exploring the Stress-Disease Connection*. Vintage Canada, 2003.
• Panda, Satchidananda. *The Circadian Code: Lose Weight, Supercharge Your Energy, and Transform Your Health from Morning to Midnight*. Rodale Books, 2018.
• Sapolsky, Robert M. *Why Zebras Don't Get Ulcers: The Acclaimed Guide to Stress, Stress-Related Diseases, and Coping*. Holt Paperbacks, 2004.
• Seaward, Brian Luke. *Managing Stress: Principles and Strategies for Health and Well-Being*. Jones & Bartlett Learning, 2017.
• Siegel, Daniel J. *The Pocket Guide to Interpersonal Neurobiology: An Integrative Handbook of the Mind*. W. W. Norton & Company, 2012.
• Stevenson, Shawn. *Sleep Smarter: 21 Essential Strategies to Sleep Your Way to a Better Body, Better Health, and Bigger Success*. Rodale Books, 2016.
• Weil, Andrew. *Spontaneous Happiness: A New Path to Emotional Well-Being*. Little, Brown Spark, 2011.

Chapter 10:
• Cuddy, Amy, et al. "Breath Control and Its Impact on the Autonomic Nervous System." *Frontiers in Human Neuroscience*, vol. 14, 2020, pp. 1–12.
• Hoffman, Martin D., and Cathy E. Fogard. "Endurance Sports and the Physiology of Breathing." *Sports Medicine*, vol. 41, no. 6, 2011, pp. 467–82.

- Jones, Andrew M., and Anni Vanhatalo. "Breathing Patterns and Oxygen Efficiency in Endurance Athletes." *European Journal of Applied Physiology*, vol. 110, no. 6, 2010, pp. 1089–98.
- McCall, Timothy. *Yoga as Medicine: The Yogic Prescription for Health and Healing*. Bantam, 2007.
- Nestor, James. *Breath: The New Science of a Lost Art*. Riverhead Books, 2020.
- Rosen, Sidney. *Qi Gong: The Secret of Youth*. Healing Tao Books, 1998.
- Stager, Joel M., and Erika B. Cordain. "Freediving and the Limits of Human Tolerance: CO_2, O_2, and Training the Breath." *Journal of Applied Physiology*, vol. 110, no. 5, 2011, pp. 1456–62.
- Swanson, Lee. *The Science of Nasal Breathing: Unlocking Endurance and Recovery*. Inner Traditions, 2019.
- Thich Nhat Hanh. *The Miracle of Mindfulness: An Introduction to the Practice of Meditation*. Beacon Press, 1975.
- Williams, Melvin H. *Nutrition for Health, Fitness, and Sport*. McGraw-Hill, 2012.

Chapter 11:
- Brown, Bessel van der Kolk. *The Body Keeps the Score: Brain, Mind, and Body in the Healing of Trauma*. Viking, 2014.
- Gabor, Maté. *When the Body Says No: Exploring the Stress-Disease Connection*. Vintage Canada, 2003.
- Levine, Peter A. *Waking the Tiger: Healing Trauma*. North Atlantic Books, 1997.
Ogden, Pat, et al. *Trauma and the Body: A Sensorimotor Approach to Psychotherapy*. W. W. Norton & Company, 2006.
- Porges, Stephen W. *The Pocket Guide to the Polyvagal Theory: The Transformative Power of Feeling Safe*. W. W. Norton & Company, 2017.
- Rothschild, Babette. *The Body Remembers: The Psychophysiology of Trauma and Trauma Treatment*. W. W. Norton & Company, 2000.
- Seigel, Daniel J. *The Developing Mind: How Relationships and the Brain Interact to Shape Who We Are*. Guilford Press, 1999.
- van der Hart, Onno, et al. *The Haunted Self: Structural Dissociation and the Treatment of Chronic Traumatization*. W. W. Norton & Company, 2006.

Chapter 12:
- Brown, Brené. *The Gifts of Imperfection: Let Go of Who You Think You're Supposed to Be and Embrace Who You Are*. Hazelden Publishing, 2010.
- Csikszentmihalyi, Mihaly. *Flow: The Psychology of Optimal Experience*. Harper Perennial Modern Classics, 2008.
- Frankl, Viktor E. *Man's Search for Meaning*. Beacon Press, 2006.
- Maté, Gabor. *When the Body Says No: Exploring the Stress-Disease Connection*. Vintage Canada, 2003.
- Rudd, Richard. *The Gene Keys: Embracing Your Higher Purpose*. Eden Press, 2013.
- Senge, Peter M., et al. *Presence: Human Purpose and the Field of the Future*. Currency, 2005.
- Siegel, Daniel J. *Mindsight: The New Science of Personal Transformation*. Bantam, 2010.

Chapter 13:

• Levine, Peter A. *Waking the Tiger: Healing Trauma*. North Atlantic Books, 1997.

• Levine, Peter A., and Maggie Kline. *Trauma Through a Child's Eyes: Awakening the Ordinary Miracle of Healing*. North Atlantic Books, 2006.

• Maté, Gabor. *When the Body Says No: Exploring the Stress-Disease Connection*. Vintage Canada, 2003.

• Naparstek, Belleruth. *Invisible Heroes: Survivors of Trauma and How They Heal*. Bantam, 2004.

• Ogden, Pat, et al. *Trauma and the Body: A Sensorimotor Approach to Psychotherapy*. W. W. Norton & Company, 2006.

• Porges, Stephen W. *The Pocket Guide to the Polyvagal Theory: The Transformative Power of Feeling Safe*. W. W. Norton & Company, 2017.

• Rothschild, Babette. *The Body Remembers: The Psychophysiology of Trauma and Trauma Treatment*. W. W. Norton & Company, 2000.

• Siegel, Daniel J. *Mindsight: The New Science of Personal Transformation*. Bantam, 2010.

van der Kolk, Bessel A. *The Body Keeps the Score: Brain, Mind, and Body in the Healing of Trauma*. Viking, 2014.

Chapter 14:

• Bjorvatn, Bjørn, et al. "The Role of Light in the Human Circadian System." *Sleep Medicine Reviews*, vol. 7, no. 1, 2003, pp. 59–72.

• Chevalier, Gaétan, et al. "Earthing: Health Implications of Reconnecting the Human Body to the Earth's Surface Electrons." *Journal of Environmental and Public Health*, vol. 2012, 2012, pp. 1–8.

• Havas, Magda. "Electromagnetic Hypersensitivity: Biological Effects of Low-Level Exposure to EMFs." *Environmental Reviews*, vol. 7, no. 2, 2000, pp. 173–204.

• Klepeis, Neil E., et al. "The National Human Activity Pattern Survey (NHAPS): A Resource for Assessing Exposure to Environmental Pollutants." *Journal of Exposure Analysis and Environmental Epidemiology*, vol. 11, no. 3, 2001, pp. 231–52.

• Lupien, Sonia J., et al. "Effects of Stress Throughout the Lifespan on the Brain, Behaviour and Cognition." *Nature Reviews Neuroscience*, vol. 10, 2009, pp. 434–45.

• Prasher, Dilip, et al. "Noise as a Public Health Problem: Emerging Evidence and Research Needs." *Environmental Health Perspectives*, vol. 117, no. 1, 2009, pp. A20–21.

• Satchidananda Panda. *The Circadian Code: Lose Weight, Supercharge Your Energy, and Transform Your Health from Morning to Midnight*. Rodale Books, 2018.

• Schneider, Marguerite, and David J. Coggon. "Physical Environment and Human Health: An Overview." *Occupational Medicine*, vol. 68, no. 3, 2018, pp. 139–44.

• Sundell, Jan. "On the History of Indoor Air Quality and Health." *Indoor Air*, vol. 14, suppl. 7, 2004, pp. 51–58.

• Zhou, Ting, et al. "Environmental Temperature and Energy Metabolism." *Journal of Physiological Sciences*, vol. 64, no. 1, 2014, pp. 19–25.

www.ingramcontent.com/pod-product-compliance
Lightning Source LLC
Chambersburg PA
CBHW081648270326
41933CB00018B/3394